THE CONCEALED REVEALED

SEARCHING FOR THE HIDDEN LYMPH NODE

by S. David Nathanson MD

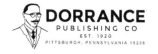

The contents of this work, including, but not limited to, the accuracy of events, people, and places depicted; opinions expressed; permission to use previously published materials included; and any advice given or actions advocated are solely the responsibility of the author, who assumes all liability for said work and indemnifies the publisher against any claims stemming from publication of the work.

All Rights Reserved
Copyright © 2021 by S. David Nathanson MD

No part of this book may be reproduced or transmitted, downloaded, distributed, reverse engineered, or stored in or introduced into any information storage and retrieval system, in any form or by any means, including photocopying and recording, whether electronic or mechanical, now known or hereinafter invented without permission in writing from the publisher.

Dorrance Publishing Co
585 Alpha Drive
Pittsburgh, PA 15238
Visit our website at *www.dorrancebookstore.com*

ISBN: 978-1-6495-7176-2
eISBN: 978-1-6495-7685-9

Endorsements

This elegantly written and totally absorbing memoir describes renowned physician-scientist Dr. Nathanson's passionate and exciting search for a hidden lymph node in breast cancer and melanoma patients. We share his scientific/medical discoveries which have eased the trauma and complications of many patients. We share and absorb his excitement of scientific discovery. Read it and you will be transported to the wondrous world of medical science and patient care at its best.

> —Michael Chopp PhD, Zolton J. Kovacs Chair in Neuroscience Research, Henry Ford Health System; Distinguished Professor, Physics, Oakland University, Rochester, MI

This delightful memoir is a wonderful window into the exciting world of biomedical research. It relates the story of Dr Nathanson's persistent fascination with lymph nodes and the lymphatic system which enabled him and others to identify the sentinel lymph node, allowing the eventual use of this new knowledge to optimize the care of breast cancer and melanoma patients world-wide.

> —Margot LaPointe PhD, Vice President for Research, Henry Ford Health System, Detroit, Michigan, USA

Doctor Nathanson's memoir is a vivid, exciting and invaluable reflection on his unique insights into the scientific discovery of the sentinel lymph node, providing the reader with a clear understanding of the fascinating world of scientific discovery that has advanced the management of breast cancer and melanoma.
—Stanley P. L. Leong, MD, FACS
Chief of Cutaneous Oncology
Center for Melanoma Research and Treatment
California Pacific Medical Center Research Institute

A succinct description of a lifelong devotion to understand how cancer spreads to lymph nodes. More important to the general reader might well be the excitement and fascination of the clinical and scientific discovery of hidden knowledge.
—Rupen Shah, MD, FACS, FSSO, Surgical Oncologist, Henry Ford Cancer Institute, Detroit, Michigan

Motivated by his patients and driven to find a better way, Dr. Nathanson shares his inspiring journey of discovery to spare cancer patients the awful fate of lymphedema, a life-altering complication of lymph node surgery for cancer. Using heart-warming stories from his own life as well as raw stories with patients whom he treated along the way, this memoir shows how basic science can improve the lives of millions.
—Timothy Padera PhD, Associate Professor, Department of Radiation Oncology, Massachusetts General Hospital, Harvard Medical School, Boston, Massachusetts, USA

A superbly written, uninhibited, wonderfully and delicately interwoven set of experiences that culminate in a gripping story of how a curious mind is transformed by a fascination with the human lymphatic system. The memoir is an example of how tenacious and repetitive enchantment with the process of discovery contributed to sentinel events that have forever changed how cancer care is delivered all over the world.

>—David Kwon MD, FACS, FSSO, System Director, Surgical Oncology & Cancer Care Pathways, Henry Ford Cancer Institute, Detroit, Michigan USA.

Contents

Acknowledgements ix
Introduction xiii
Chapter 1. Lymph Node Metastasis 1
Chapter 2. A New Word 13
Chapter 3. Curiosity and Creativity 17
Chapter 4. Hodgkin's Disease 25
Chapter 5. Splenomegaly 33
Chapter 6. Lymphadenopathy 45
Chapter 7. Anatomy 51
Chapter 8. Darwin and the Unseen 61
Chapter 9. Seeing 67
Chapter 10. Advanced Learning 75
Chapter 11. The Immune System 81
Chapter 12. Seeing the Hidden 87
Chapter 13. Eyes Wide Open 93
Chapter 14. Westwood Bound 99
Chapter 15. Lymphedema 105
Chapter 16. Principal Investigator 113
Chapter 17. Unravelling Lymph Node Metastasis 123
Chapter 18. The Sentinel Node in Melanoma 131
Chapter 19. Paraguay and the Sentinel Node 137
Chapter 20. On the Shoulders of Giants 143
Chapter 21. A Surgical Revolution Unfolds 149
Chapter 22. The Metal Clip 157
Chapter 23. The Concealed Is Revealed 163

Acknowledgements

People, places, and events have influenced my career and encouraged me to write this story of the discovery of the sentinel lymph node biopsy and my role in the discovery.

There are so many people to thank, some departed, some alive, that I would have to add dozens of pages of names if I were to thank them individually. Suffice it to say, many of them appear in my book, and it is easy to tell who influenced me greatly, and I'm very grateful that they took the time and devoted the energy to my education and knowledge.

There are many people in my current work life at Henry Ford Health System, where I've been a senior surgical oncologist for thirty-eight years, who deserve a lot of credit for helping me achieve my clinical and research goals. Amongst those are Margot La Pointe, PhD, director of research, a brilliant researcher and administrator, who helped me with ideas and research space and encouraged me to pursue the difficult life of a physician-scientist; Michael Chopp, PhD, a physicist by training, who has become one of the world's pre-eminent neuroscientists, a friend whose unrelenting optimism, scientific vigor, and beautiful spirit helped me overcome many frustrating failed laboratory experiments; Scott Dulchavsky, MD, PhD, the chairman of surgery, who came to understand why I, a surgeon, should be so motivated by deep biologic questions and a relentless need to solve them and whose understanding was vital to my success; Kasty Karvelis, MD, chief of nuclear medicine, who unquestioningly supported my restless urge to do the first sentinel node biopsies in Michigan; Richard Zarbo, MD, chairman of pathology, a staunch friend and ally who provided the vital pathologic support for the sentinel node era; Eleanor Walker, MD, radiation oncologist, a colleague and friend who helped promote the new era of the sentinel node; Kenneth Levin, MD, radiation oncologist, a colleague and friend whose need for high quality breast cancer treatments mirrors my own. I thank the many other colleagues who staunchly supported my efforts at introducing new ideas into our oncologic practice including: Randa Loutfi, MD; Haythem Ali, MD; David Kwon, MD; Rupen Shah, MD; Lynne Wachna, BS, RN; Cathie Smith, BS, RN; many medical oncologists and generations of surgical trainees that I taught and who have gone off into the world to their own practices. My research collaborators, assistants, and statisticians were all vital to my sentinel node studies.

Don Morton, MD, mentor, teacher, and friend left us in 2014 but not before he established himself as the pioneer of the sentinel node biopsy in melanoma. He is a legend in the world of surgical oncology and a giant in my life. Without him, I might have ended up homeless on the streets of Los Angeles. I continue to seek the sentinel node because of him.

Much of my scientific writings about sentinel nodes were vigorously supported by Stanley Leong, MD in San Francisco who tirelessly promoted the importance of the concept of the hidden node at international meetings that he set up and the editing of many books about the subject to which I contributed.

It may sound strange to thank the COVID-19 pandemic, but without the time I was forced to take away from work, I may not have written this book. My hope is that the infectious scourge disappears soon, and I am so sorry for the families that have lost loved ones.

I had a lot of help from Perdita Finn, my editor in New York, who helped mold the contents of this book in firm but supportive ways.

Susan Leitman, PhD supported me throughout the writing of the book, rigorously reading every chapter, suggesting changes, recognizing stories that might not fit, and gently urging me forward when I needed that.

Finally, to the thousands of patients who took the chance with an unproven technique, the brave men and women who agreed to help me accumulate one of the largest databases on sentinel nodes in the country, thank you!

Introduction

Lymph, unlike blood, is a clear fluid generated from the circulatory system in the tissues of the body. Blood is red and is easily seen in blood vessels while lymph, carried by a large network of tiny lymphatic vessels to the nearest lymph nodes, in clusters in the neck, armpit, groins, and a few other places, is invisible to the naked eye, even to operating surgeons. The lymph fluid passes through multiple lymph nodes and eventually passes back into the blood stream.

Lymph nodes are small, solid, kidney-shaped structures that survey the lymph passing through them and filter foreign infectious organisms, like bacteria and viruses, producing an immune response, that mostly protects us from sometimes lethal damage.

Cancers affecting body structures, like the breast, tend to metastasize to the regional lymph nodes, a process first recognized only within the last two hundred years by clinicians and pathologists. The first operations designed to cure patients with breast cancer were developed in the late nineteenth century. Recognizing the frequency of regional lymph node metastasis, surgeons began doing the operation of radical mastectomy by removing the entire breast, all the lymph nodes in the armpit, and the tissues between them, including the pectoral muscles, a devastating procedure with long term complications, including marked swelling of the arm, or lymphedema. This cosmetically unattractive effect also resulted in functionally and emotionally difficult days for the patients, forced to adapt to a new bodily image and to spend hours every day trying to live "normally." The arm could swell to gigantic proportions making it almost impossible to dress in normal clothes, and women were forced to adapt their lifestyles around clothing that not only hid the deformity but were reconstructed to allow them to put their arms into shirts with large sleeves or into blouses with enlarged arm holes. For decades the mastectomy was the standard operation to treat breast cancer and physicians advocated it while women tolerated the discomfort, accepting the possibility of lymphedema, because there were no alternative treatments and about one third of the patients were cured by the procedure. I remember as a young surgeon in training my first encounters with patients struggling daily with life dealing with lymphedema and not truly understanding their grievances. But I changed as I began to understand the hardships that patients encountered.

Lymphedema also rendered patients susceptible to potentially lethal infections starting in the swollen limb, and many women succumbed to cellulitis and the resulting septicemia before antibiotics were used in the 1940s. People died from the side effects of the operation even when they were cured of their cancers. Even now, when many types of antibiotics are available, patients with blood poisoning starting in lymphedematous limbs often require lengthy, expensive, and uncomfortable hospital stays.

Melanoma is another malignant tumor that is sometimes treated by removing all the regional lymph nodes with resultant lymphedema. In this disease the lymph nodes in the armpit may be removed, just like in breast cancer, and patients are just as likely to get swollen arms as those patients in whom the operation is done for breast cancer. Melanoma may also occur in parts of the body where the nodes that need to be removed are in the groin, and patients in whom groin and adjacent pelvic lymph nodes are removed are even more likely to get gigantic swelling of the legs, requiring lifelong daily efforts to limit the swelling by physical therapy, massage, bandaging, elastic stockings, and external electrical pumps, all of which are time-consuming, costly, uncomfortable, and limiting.

I encountered the lymphatic system as a young child and then repeatedly as I grew older and went to medical school and trained in surgery, where I first encountered patients who had tumors that had spread to lymph nodes. I became incurably curious about this aggressive behavior of some tumors, and my research career matured as I asked more and more questions about this phenomenon. My story would probably not have developed any further towards research in lymph node metastasis if I had not also been inquisitive and immersed myself into discovering new ways to do things. Not that I was in any way unique because we all have a propensity to investigate new ways of living, and everyone has their own way to improve the world while seeking happiness.

My first serious laboratory experiments as a twenty-year-old medical student were a continuation of serendipitous events that I can now look back upon when trying to understand how new ideas came to me and how I was lucky enough to bring new ideas into medicine. Medicine is a profession that encourages knowledge of hundreds of thousands of facts which we physicians learn to cram into our heads at a relatively young age. However, it takes years of experience to understand how those facts connect to the patients we are privileged to treat. Young medical students and doctors, like apprentices, are steered through the process of connecting the facts and understanding diseases and how to manage them by wise teachers who we follow.

Louis Pasteur, the great nineteenth century French scientist, is reputed to have said that "discovery favors the prepared mind." Detailed knowledge of any subject is crucial to anyone seeking to explore the boundaries of knowledge and to discover new insights. Some of the knowledge that led me to explore the lymph nodes in cancer came directly from textbooks and scientific articles published in the literature, some from my teachers and professors, and some from patients and friends. A friend made me question the standard operations to remove the regional lymph nodes in breast cancer because she had severe, life-altering lymphedema following a radical mastectomy as a young woman. Talking to her and listening to her concerns and seeing the extensive daily routines she went through in order to live a reasonable life prepared my mind for finding a way to avoid doing the operation she and many other people had, although it took many years of experiments and clinical practice for me to get there.

There are many ways of observing. Snakes use infrared vision, elephants can sense low frequency sound that humans cannot hear, and turtles can sense magnetic fields, but we humans all walk through life aware only of those things we can see, hear, touch, smell, and taste. Occasionally, we also imagine things without using those five senses, ideas that come to us through reading or through discussions with others or by observing something new that we hadn't seen before. But we all know that there are many things that exist around us that we can't see or experience through our usual senses. We've all came to understand this truth recently with the COVID-19 pandemic, understanding that there is an invisible enemy around us that can cause a serious disease. My experience operating on patients with melanoma, breast or other cancers was somewhat similar when it came to the lymphatic vessels. I knew they were there because scientists in the lab had exposed them by injecting chemical substances, like mercury, that filled them and made them visible. But they weren't visible without some kind of injection. Confronted by a question that needed addressing in the lab I came up with ways to see the lymphatic vessels and would allow me to see the pathway from tumors to the first lymph node that the cancerous cells would enter. Any advances in science, the elaboration of new ideas, need essential and sequential steps to be in place before one can hope for important changes to occur.

New ideas that change the way we practice medicine have grown at an exponential rate in the past fifty years, and most of those ideas have come from multiple sources. It is not as common in the modern era compared to the past to find a new idea that came from one person. One only must look at the Nobel Prizes in Medicine and Physiology where we often see two or three people awarded the prize every year, sometimes because they worked together, and sometimes because two or more people had the same idea and worked independently. We all need to honor the giants that came before us, as Isaac Newton first intoned when he recognized that he could not have produced his groundbreaking ideas in physics, mathematics, and astronomy without standing on the shoulders of those giants who came before him. So, too, I'm indelibly indebted to mentors and supporters that helped me find a new way to recognize a vitally important lymph node.

The sentinel lymph node, initially both theoretically and physically hidden from view, has emerged from its hiding place. The new operation of removing only the sentinel lymph node in breast cancer and melanoma has revolutionized surgical treatment, saved hundreds of thousands of patients the agony of removing all the lymph nodes, and has so far saved the health care system in the United States an estimated seven billion dollars.

The lymph system is very old, and nothing about it has changed in humans. In this memoir, I show how our understanding has changed as we have discovered what was formerly concealed, the sentinel node, one of several regional lymph nodes to which cancer spreads from primary organs, such as the breast, skin, stomach, colon, pancreas, and lungs.

Chapter 1

Lymph Node Metastasis

Howard, a well-known entertainment lawyer with offices in Century City, and his wife, Judy, were anxious to understand how he had developed an enlarged lymph node in his right groin filled with metastatic melanoma, a darkly pigmented skin cancer that sometimes spreads to lymph nodes. Dressed in a light brown suit with a red tie, the anxious, blonde-haired, blue-eyed, light-skinned, middle-aged man with a noticeable nystagmus, repetitive, uncontrolled side to side, up and down, or circular pattern movements of both eyes, was in the clinic to see my chief, Doctor Donald Morton, an internationally renowned melanoma expert.

My role as a fellow training to become a surgical oncologist at UCLA in Los Angeles was to fully evaluate the patient before calling Morton to see him in the clinic. A dermatologist had found no evidence of melanoma in the skin of his right leg or lower abdomen or back or anywhere else and had referred the patient to Morton as "melanoma of unknown primary origin," a condition where melanoma had spread to a lymph node and where a careful search in the usual anatomic areas where the melanoma may have originated revealed normal skin and no prior history of a treated pigmented lesion.

Lymph nodes dominated my daily life for the three years of my specialized post-graduate training in surgical oncology. Every patient with melanoma, or breast cancer, or cancers of other organs, from the thyroid gland in the neck, or the pancreas, or the stomach, or the colon could potentially spread to the lymph nodes closest to that organ, important information for the surgical oncologist treating the patient because it would determine the treatment and the stage of the disease. In 1979 the way for me to determine whether a melanoma had metastasized to the regional lymph nodes was by palpation. A melanoma in the leg could spread to the lymph nodes in the ipsilateral groin, and I examined the patients with melanomas by feeling for enlarged lumps with a firm consistency in the area where lymph nodes normally grouped together. In Howard's case, there did not seem to be a primary melanoma in the skin that could account for the malignant disease in the groin lymph node.

Puzzled by this unusual presentation, I used an ultraviolet lamp on the skin of the trunk and legs to look for an area that might be invisible to the human eye with normal light but might show changes associated with a prior melanoma that had regressed or disappeared because of a spontaneous reaction to the melanoma by the patient's own immune system. This examination also showed nothing unusual. The patient had no history of melanoma in the past, but he remembered having a pigmented lesion removed from his left eye when at Harvard Law School in the 1950s.

"Was that a melanoma in your eye?" I asked.

"No. They told me it was benign."

I called the Massachusetts Eye and Ear Infirmary in Boston to ask if they could retrieve the tissue slides from twenty years previously, and they agreed to send them to me by Federal Express.

I knocked on Morton's door to tell him about the patient.

His high-pitched voice with a slight Southern brogue seemed incongruous emanating from his large frame, comfortably covered by an immaculate white coat, his name emblazoned in blue above the pocket. If I had met him and he had said nothing, I would have imagined him to have a deep baritone voice. If I had heard the voice without seeing him, I would have guessed that he was a small guy, a little nerdy, tentative and slow, perhaps a little unsure of himself. But there it was, the slow and deliberate voice emanating from the legendary chief of Surgical Oncology at UCLA, a man of humble beginnings in rural Richwood, West Virginia, a small coal-mining town tucked away in the Appalachians, who had grown up dirt poor during the Great Depression, the son of a coal miner, reared in a house built by his father with no electricity or indoor plumbing, who had tended pigs, cows, and chickens in the morning before school, and then again after school, completing his household chores before he was allowed to do his homework by the light of a kerosene lamp.

How could a man with that kind of upbringing, a man only nine years older than me, have achieved such a high standing in the academic world of surgical oncology? I had come to experience his grit, determination, confidence, wisdom, knowledge, understanding, and infectious optimism while working side by side as a surgical oncology fellow with him for three years. As I got to know him better, he confided in me that he overcame the limitations of poverty because of his supportive mother who recognized his sharp mind and intense intellect and encouraged him to enroll in Berea College in Kentucky, which provided free education to qualified students from poor families. It must have been quite a transformation for him to move out west and complete an undergraduate degree at the University of California, Berkeley, and then cross the Bay and complete his medical degree and surgical training at UCSF, interrupted briefly by fellowship training at the National Cancer Institute.

Morton had begun to revolutionize surgical oncology when he returned to the NCI as a senior surgeon, where he eventually headed the tumor immunology section and where his observations of spontaneous remissions in melanoma ignited his lifelong dedication and interest in immunotherapy, surgical oncology, and melanoma.

I took the chief to see Howard and told him about the unusual presentation, the unique way in which he had developed a melanoma metastasis in a groin lymph node without an obvious primary melanoma in the leg, or lower trunk, or perineum.

After seeing Howard and speaking to Judy, Morton and I sat in his office to discuss what to do with this strange case.

"What do you think we should do with him?" Morton asked.

"Well, I guess it depends upon whether we believe this is an unknown primary melanoma or not. If it is, he would be a candidate for a radical right inguino-pelvic lymphadenectomy. I'm not sure what I would do if the slides from Boston show that he had an eye melanoma in his twenties as a law student. Can melanomas from the eye metastasize to lymph nodes in the groin? Have you ever seen that?"

"Melanomas can spread to distant lymph nodes through the blood stream," he said. "That is very uncommon. Let's do some scans and X-rays to see if he has melanoma anywhere else. Where does eye melanoma usually metastasize?"

I remembered *Bailey and Love*, my surgery text book, a beloved reference of many surgical trainees from the British Commonwealth countries of the United Kingdom, West Indies, Kenya, Uganda, Ghana, Canada, India, Pakistan, Australia, New Zealand, South Africa, and about forty other countries, and I could see in my mind's eye a picture of a jaundiced man with a protuberant belly and an empty eye socket with a caption that read: *"Beware of the man with the glass eye and enlarged liver."*

"To the liver," I replied.

"Yes, and melanoma from anywhere in the body can spread to the liver, although it usually goes to lymph nodes first. Eye melanomas tend to go straight to the liver, without traveling to the lymph nodes."

Alistair Cochran, a world-renowned melanoma pathologist at UCLA, reviewed Howard's iris tumor from the 1950s and declared that it was a melanoma. The groin lymph node showed melanoma. Eye melanomas that seem cured after surgical removal of the lesion may show up as metastases to the liver many years later, but I found no similar case of metastasis to peripheral lymph nodes in the reported cases in the world. Even lymph nodes in the neck, where skin melanomas of the head and neck region metastasize, are not sites where eye melanomas metastasize. Because of this observation, Morton advised the patient to have all the lymph nodes removed from his right groin and the lower part of his pelvis and told him he probably had a melanoma in the right leg which had spontaneously disappeared and was no longer visible.

I returned to the examining room to talk to Howard and Judy filled with doubt about the wisdom of doing the procedure that Morton had suggested because I had seen so many patients in whom this operation had caused the long-term complication of lymphedema, swelling of the leg that required daily management with massage, frequent bandaging, wearing of a cumbersome elastic stocking, and the nighttime use of a noisy and uncomfortable external pressure pump.

"Do you agree that I should have this operation?" he asked.

"It is pretty standard, and Doctor Morton does it well," I said.

"What can I expect to happen?"

"The operation is done under general anesthetic, and you will need to stay in the hospital for about five days. You will have an incision from here to here." I pointed to the anatomic site of the incision.

"Will I be able to walk?"

"Initially, you will need to stay in bed for two days and not walk. If the incision is healing well, you will be able to walk a little on the third day with the help of a physical therapist. Once you go home, we will give you instructions about how to limit movement of your right hip."

"Is there a problem with the healing in the groin?"

"A small percentage of people develop what we call wound edge necrosis, where there is insufficient blood supply to the incision site, and there is a danger that it can open up and dead tissue develop in that area."

"Is that a problem?"

"It can be a problem. The lymph nodes that are removed are embedded in fat which normally protects the major blood vessels to your leg. When they're removed, the only tissue covering the blood vessels is skin and some fat under the skin. If that area opens because of wound edge necrosis, there is nothing to protect the blood vessels, and an infection in that area could be dangerous, perhaps resulting in rupture of the blood vessels."

"That doesn't sound good. How often does that terrible complication happen?"

"I've not seen it happen to our patients, but it is described in the textbooks."

"Are there other complications that I should know about?"

I told him about the chronic leg swelling.

"That sounds bad. Do you have data that clearly justifies this operation in my case?"

Because Howard's presentation was so extraordinary, I could not calculate the likelihood of additional node metastases when one lymph node in the groin tested positive for melanoma because that type of calculation required me to use numbers from Morton's own database, or from data around the world, and such data was not available for patients in whom the melanoma originated in the eye. I felt that the likelihood of him having additional lymph nodes with metastatic melanoma would be very small. I shared this information with Howard and told him about my own concerns regarding the value of removing all the lymph nodes, especially since no one had adequately studied the outcome of patients undergoing complete removal of all the lymph nodes, a radical lymphadenectomy, compared to those patients whose lymph nodes were left intact. I knew that leaving the lymph nodes intact would probably leave him free of limb swelling but admitted that I didn't know for certain that removing all the nodes was beneficial.

"I'm not sure what to do," said Howard, looking at Judy who seemed confused.

"Morton is a world authority on this disease, and I think I would do what he recommends," I said.

Howard and Judy discussed the options and decided to do the operation.

Surgical removal of the lymph nodes from the groin is a beautiful procedure, exposing gleaming anatomic details that reminded me of my days teaching anatomy to medical students in Johannesburg. I spent a few hours before Howard's planned surgery reviewing Tobias's textbook of human anatomy and familiarizing myself with the relationships amongst the muscles, fascia, nerves, blood vessels, and lymph nodes, preparing myself mentally for the operation. Preparation for the emotional side of the surgery was easy because I loved the way an unhurried Morton, standing on the opposite side of the operating table, gently coaxed me through each step, hundreds of coordinated movements designed to progressively separate the lymph nodes, embedded in fat and connective tissues, from the functionally important structures to be left behind. I was not always comfortable operating with other attending surgeons on the other side of the table when they wanted to get the process over with quickly, rushing as if they were in some competitive sporting activity, finding that unsettling and often quite dangerous. My metabolic rhythm fitted well with Morton and made the operation even more appealing.

My mind, now in my eleventh year since graduating from medical school, and with at least nine of those years spent operating on patients, was quite comfortable thinking about all sorts of ideas while my hands maneuvered dissecting instruments, cauterized tissues to stop bleeding, tied larger blood vessels with sutures, avoided injury to normal tissues that would be left intact, and sowed tissues together. In Howard's case, I thought repeatedly about the decision to remove all these lymph nodes, remembering many patients who had developed chronic lymphedema of the leg after this procedure. I wasn't sure we were doing the right operation. I wasn't sure whether he needed an operation at all. Those thoughts were enhanced when the pathologist found no more tumor in the twenty-five lymph nodes that we removed.

I couldn't help remembering the TV commercial for a popular vegetable juice where the actor gently hit his forehead with his hand and said: "I could have had a V8!" *If we had only not removed all these groin lymph nodes*, I thought. *What good will it do him now, and we can't put those nodes back.* Now Howard would be condemned to wearing a thick elastic stocking for the rest of his life, putting it on every morning and taking it off every night, trying to prevent it from rolling down by using suspenders, and an uncomfortable girdle, laundering it every second night, replacing it every three months with a new one, possibly having to use an external pump on his leg at night, and making extra sure that he didn't injure the skin of the leg in any way, including when cutting his toe nails so as to prevent infection.

As the junior member of the team taking care of Howard, it was my job to see him in the hospital every day for five days after his surgery until he was ready to be discharged home and to make sure he had all his needs met. Every time I walked into his hospital room, I thought about how he might have avoided the expense and discomfort of the operation, the anesthetic, the bandages and dressings, the daily antiseptic painting of his skin, the medications with their potential side effects, the plastic tube that drained the surgical site for three weeks until it was removed, the days away from his family and from his busy law practice, the clamor and bustle of the busy nurses and doctors, the excess noise of janitors cleaning floors and walls and other surfaces, the repeated loud talking of visitors and students, woken to have his temperature and blood pressure taken or to be given a sleeping pill, or by a kitchen help bringing a tray of food, or the physical therapist coming to help him walk around the floor. If only we had rethought this whole process and accepted that he represented the rare case where his eye melanoma had metastasized to a single right groin lymph node, a unique event not previously reported, so rare that it was very unlikely that other lymph nodes in the groin or pelvis would have metastases.

I didn't share my questions and concerns about the value of his procedure, but I saw Howard and Judy often in the clinic over the next few weeks, and later, after they invited me to visit them at home, this charming, boisterous man and I shared a lot of personal thoughts and ideas, especially when he received monthly treatments with a concoction containing altered tuberculosis bacteria, bacillus Calmette-Guerin, or BCG, injected into the skin of the lower abdomen and upper truncal areas on both sides of the body, a method devised by Morton to stimulate the regional lymph nodes in the groin and armpit and thought to kickstart the immune system to work against melanoma in the body.

BCG, shown to inhibit the growth of tumors in hamsters, and to induce non-specific immune responses in rodents and in human controls, had interested Morton when he was in the surgery branch at the National Cancer Institute, and he loved to show us pictures of a patient whom he had treated with hundreds of recurrent melanomas in the skin of her arm. Injecting BCG directly into selected small tumors made them disappear, and some of the other skin melanomas close by that had not been injected also regressed, suggesting an immune response. I could understand the rationale for injecting BCG into Howard since there was no other treatment that worked in melanoma at the time, but Morton had no proof that it worked in patients when the vaccine was injected into the skin and not directly into the melanoma.

I was reminded of Peter Medawar, Nobel laureate, whom I had met in England, and my basic scientist friends in the immunology department at UCLA, who would have questioned the use of BCG in anybody other than children in India where it produced immunity to tuberculosis, a devastating disease in many third world countries. I wondered when Morton would do a randomized prospective study in melanoma patients at high risk of recurrence where half the patients would receive BCG vaccinations and half would receive a placebo. But he was so convinced of its value and so committed to saving as many patients as possible that we all did his bidding with intense conviction, treating hundreds of patients with metastatic melanoma.

The intensity of a conviction that a hypothesis is true has no bearing on whether it is true or not. Eventually, faulty hypotheses are excusable claiming they will be superseded in due course by better ones, but they can do grave harm to patients who are drawn in by the clinician, like Morton, who has fallen deeply in love with the hypothesis and unwilling to believe that it might be defective. For some reason Morton was initially unwilling to expose his hypothesis to the critical clinical study until years later. But the importance of his conviction that immunotherapy, of which BCG was one of the first and quite primitive, would eventually prove to be effective in melanoma has proven to be true. In the second decade of the twenty-first century, James Allison received a Nobel Prize for producing effective immunotherapy for melanomas and other cancers.

Any clinical scientist, like Morton, who is inventive and imaginative, is likely to make mistakes over matters of interpretation, likely, that is, to take a wrong view or propound a hypothesis that does not stand up to criticism. That kind of mistake is not intentionally harmful, and it is part of the turmoil of scientific life, and it is quite common in clinical science for physicians to hold strong ideas that are later proven wrong. Morton had a large, well-funded BCG program, and I was convinced there was likely to be a positive effect of the vaccine in patients like Howard because the theory seemed to point in that direction. I took part in the process of recommending BCG to patients, and that's what I had done with Howard, vigorously participating in a treatment that Morton was forced to eventually put to the true scientific test and was eventually shown to be ineffective for patients like Howard. Human nature is such that a clinician admitting such a mistake, as Morton did years later, without trying to lay down a voluminous smoke screen to conceal the error, might even gain credit for such a declaration.

I wanted Howard to survive his metastatic melanoma but neither the radical operation nor the intense non-specific BCG vaccination nor my repeated prayers could keep away the angel of death from this wonderful man. Six months after I left Morton's group and moved to Pleasant Hill, Contra Costa County, to do more surgical training at the Martinez Veterans Administration Hospital nearby, Howard and Judy came to visit on their way to Oregon to do white water rafting with their children on one of the rivers there. He had been well, and his care was managed by Morton and a new surgical oncology fellow. Late that night, he had intense pain in the liver area because of liver metastases from his eye melanoma. His severely swollen right leg was covered by the partially effective elastic stocking. There was no treatment that I could give him other than some mild analgesics, and he went back home the next day to see Morton. There was no effective treatment, and a few months later, he died, unwilling to give up even at the very end, after a valiant fight which I saw directly because I was visiting Los Angeles for a wedding and saw him at home.

My invaluable time with Morton gave me further insight into both the practice of surgical oncology and the need for clinical, basic science and translational studies in trying to improve the treatment of patients with solid tumors of the breast, skin, soft tissues, stomach, colon, rectum, liver, pancreas, and the endocrine glands of the neck, abdomen, and chest. My mind was filled with my years at UCLA as I drove north on highway 101 to start the final phases of my surgical training in the San Francisco Bay Area, reflecting on how I had learned to think seriously about different types of scientific and clinical endeavors.

What way could I spend the rest of my career improving knowledge? I was imbued with the scientific spirit, and I knew I could do scientific research with more vigor and understanding than before my UCLA experience. Anyone can, by patient experimentation, see what happens if you add this or another substance in proportion, and using variable conditions, vary the experiment in any number of ways, something every baker knows and uses to make a better cake. I wanted to be more like Galileo, doing critical experiments, not so much to prove that anything was true but rather to refute the opposite idea that it might not be true. My experience of human fallibility in the past five years had taught me that scientists should state that their hypotheses were (or were not) consistent with the hypothesis under investigation. I had learned from my exposure to graduate doctoral students at UCLA that my prior way of thinking, the clinical deductive reasoning of surgical research, did not always clearly focus on limited variables and therefore might have diluted or swayed the "truth."

The idea that kept coming up, the idea that might keep me busy for the rest of my career, was the recurring thought that there must be a way of discerning whether a melanoma or breast cancer had metastasized to a regional node or not.

That is what drove me forward to do studies that eventually changed the world of surgical oncology.

Chapter 2

A New Word

Early on in my childhood I wanted to do many things myself. One burning desire from an early age was to visit my father's business without him driving me there. In those days, it was not unusual for an eleven-year-old boy to explore the noisy, energetic city of Johannesburg on his own, even though it required walking alone through some rough neighborhoods.

One afternoon after elementary school, I took the municipal bus from my parents' house in Yeoville, a suburb of Johannesburg, to the downtown terminal. It promised to be an adventure, and I gave myself a task that required careful planning, making sure I took the correct bus at the right time and paying for the trip with a book of coupons that I bought with my own pocket money. After studying a map of downtown Johannesburg, I had planned to walk about a mile to my father's business, carefully noting the street names. Walking south and west, I discovered the Johannesburg City Library, about halfway between the bus terminal and my father's business.

Here, in the middle of downtown Johannesburg, the largest city in South Africa, was a large building with a massive and imposing triple-arch with metal doors on which were carved "LJ" and "BJ" for the English "Library of Johannesburg" and the Afrikaans "Biblioteek Johannesburg." On the sides of the building, the one closest to Pritchard Street and the opposite side closest to Fox Street, were face statues and larger statues around the building of what I later came to understand belonged to great literary, historical, scientific, and philosophical figures.

I walked in to the library, intrigued with the idea of books and reading, which I loved, intending to explore a little, maybe to see what it felt like to be in a very large room where shelves were filled with many books, and then to continue my journey to my dad's gas station; I entered the quiet, solid grey building. Uncertain that I would know where to go and convinced that someone would yell at me because I didn't know enough to be there on my own, I was relieved when the librarian did not even look at me as I examined the layout of the first floor, exploring the book-laden shelves scattered throughout the large space. I was the youngest person in the building.

I had learned to read in Mrs. Barnett's kindergarten, where the teacher encouraged me to put my index finger under the word on the open page and say it out loud and move to the next word.

"The cat ate the rat."

It felt so good each time I successfully read what the teacher asked. What a thrill to recognize, read, and understand the sentences! School books were not enough for me, and soon, starting in the first grade, I had my own books at home. My parents were thrilled that I liked to read, and they often gave me books as presents. Most recently I had read every new *Hardy Boys* and *Captain Biggles* mystery, and adventure stories filled with swashbuckling, sword-carrying heroes from the European Continent, and gun-toting cowboys from the American West. I developed a rich imagery, often daydreaming, imagining myself to be one of the characters in the books, and dreaming colorful, hero-filled dreams at night.

Holding a book in my hands, attracted by its cover, design, or binding, turning the pages and feeling the texture, smelling the unique book scent, admiring the beauty of the typeface, and feeling the stories welling up and outwards, often creating visual images of people, places, events, and relationships, was (and still is) a thrilling experience. Those were the days of secret gratification of reading a book under the covers by flashlight after "lights out." When I opened a book, I anticipated the excitement of discovering stories, and I loved the power I felt of being in charge. Unlike the movies, when I sat in a theater, watching the characters and the narrative arc develop, where I had no control over when I could stop and think about the style and shape of the story and not revisit a part I really wanted to explore more deeply, I could decide when to open and close my book or to reread a passage that I didn't quite understand. I was the one who decided on the pacing. I could stop or keep going, linger over a phrase and restart. I merely sampled most books, completed others, and completely and thoroughly consumed only a few. Those were the few that drew me in, grabbed hold of every sense, immersed me in imaginary realities, populated my conversations and enriched my dreams. When entirely captivated by a book, I wasn't bored, and time flew by, making me feel refreshed, relaxed, and nourished, as satisfied with my day as I might have felt after eating chocolate ice cream.

How different from my collection the books on the vast bookshelves looked that day in the public library. They looked old and important. Most of them were leather or cloth-bound, in different colors, some black, others brown, some green or yellow or burgundy. The titles, printed on the spine and front cover in gold, black, white, or silver, were often big words that I didn't understand. That didn't stop me from looking through the books that seemed inviting.

I pretended that I knew the meaning of the title as I pulled a book out. The book next to it came out as well and fell on the floor. As I leaned forward to retrieve the book that had dropped, I noticed a picture on the open page. Looking at it drew me inexorably to turn the page and look at other pictures. I was intrigued and took the book to a reading table and sat down to examine it more carefully.

The pictures in the book were photographs and diagrams, and they fascinated me even though I didn't know exactly what they meant. The words were intriguing. "Anatomy" was one that I didn't quite understand, but I wrote it down on a piece of paper, so I could look it up in the dictionary at home. "Physiology was another that I'd never heard. What did that mean? It didn't matter. I just continued to read the complex words, not understanding what I read, until I came to a story that I could understand. Not quite like the stories I was used to reading, but at least it was a story that came from Greek and

Roman times. I knew about stories from those ancient days because my classes at school included Greek mythology and the story of Romulus and Remus and the mythical origins of the seven hills of Rome.

It seems there was a creature whose name was "Nymph" that lived in clear streams and rivers and a Roman god "Lympha," whose name meant "clear spring water." The fluid in the lymphatic system was clear whereas blood was red. This book was about lymph, and I had learned a new word.

I put the book back on the shelf and walked the remaining few blocks to meet my father, and I was excited to tell him about lymph and lymphatics.

Chapter 3

Curiosity and Creativity

Little boys, often full of mischief, curious and imaginative, cognitively flexible, ready to take risks, and while not necessarily intellectually brilliant or socially mature, often come up with ideas that originate almost entirely within them. Parents and teachers can celebrate and encourage such behavior while gently guiding the children in their endeavors, overseeing their successes and empathizing with their failures. My insatiable curiosity, coupled with a need to find something new and valuable, was supported by my parents and teachers and enabled me to learn how to do experiments at an early age.

My friend Colin and I, fresh and excited by ideas, tried out new things every day, notions that most often excited the frustration of our parents, teachers, and, sometimes, our own classmates.

But sometimes we came up with concepts that worked well and startled our parents, who smiled at how smart we were, and then proudly boasted to everyone in the neighborhood as if they had produced young, resourceful, obviously original and inventive geniuses.

One of my crazy ideas resulted in my lifelong passion for photography and my love of experiments.

Learning to use my Kodak Brownie box camera 6-20 at age six was one of my first experiments. Taking three-inch pictures required me to choose my light and subject carefully, look in the range finder, make sure the sun was behind while moving my angle to avoid seeing my shadow in the picture, correct for parallax, compensate for where the top of the head appeared in the image, hold my breath, press the button to take the picture while keeping the camera still, and advance the film. Later, I would call those "variables" in my experiments.

Waiting a week for the drug store to develop my black and white film took what seemed like forever. Tearing open the carefully sealed envelope, like a ravenous dog chomping on a fresh steak, I carefully examined each picture, noting mistakes in composition, lighting, and exposure. My pictures did get better, but I knew that there had to be a better way for me to learn photography. I needed a teacher, or a book, or both, to make better pictures.

Colin and I met at my house after school when we were in the fourth grade at the local elementary school. While running around in the back yard kicking the soccer ball to each other, I yelled: "Do you think we can learn how to develop and print black and white pictures that we take with our cameras?"

"You're crazy," he yelled.

"Why?"

"Do you know how to do it?"

"Oh, I don't know. Maybe we can get a book and read how to do it."

"I think we should ask my dad. Maybe he knows."

So, Colin asked his dad. He didn't think we were old enough. Besides, it was too expensive. I asked my parents, and they said the same to me.

The next time I picked up my pictures from the drug store, I saw a book on photography on one of the shelves. It was a big book with lots of pictures and chapters on how to use the camera and on how to develop and print from black and white film. It looked complicated, but I was determined to try it out. My birthday was six months away, but my father agreed to buy me the book. I fondly remember this activity now as I think about starting a new experiment in my lab.

Whenever I had a new book to read, I would excuse myself after dinner, close my bedroom door, and sit comfortably at a small wooden desk, turn on the lamp, and start reading.

When what appears on the page suddenly lights up in one's mind, the joy of understanding is almost better than fresh watermelon on a hot summer day. I immediately connected with the ideas in the photography book, and I took those ideas and thoughts out with me when I pointed my camera on walks in the neighborhood. I captured three-dimensional effects on two-dimensional surfaces when I used the vanishing point ideas of Renaissance paintings, ideas originating from architecture and the designs of buildings and first used by artists in 14th century Italy. I saw my pictures of gardens, schoolyards, soccer fields, neighborhood shops, and the family come alive. I loved the chapter on portraits because I learned to focus on facial features and to place the camera in a Goldilocks position so as not to distort the image or to lose details—not too far and not too near. I used toy cars and dolls to do tabletop photography.

Buying photographic chemicals and their containers for developing black and white film was exciting. I found a photography store in Hillbrow, a suburb close to our home, and slowly, much too slowly for me, over a few months, I collected glass bottles, chemicals, funnels, photographic paper, tongs, a contact printer, a thermometer, a red safety light, a stop watch, and, finally, a black plastic developing tank. Years later, when directing lab research as a physician-scientist, I used these learned habits and remembered how to create situations that allowed me to ask probing questions.

Colin and I did our first experiments in printing from negatives in the living room at home. After covering the living room windows with thick blankets to make the room dark, we took a negative, a portrait of my father, and, using the red safety light, took out one piece of unexposed photographic paper from the light-proof box, placed it in the contact printer with the glossy side next to the negative, and turned on the light to expose the paper. From reading the book, we knew that it mattered how long the light was on and how bright the light bulb inside.

After twenty seconds of exposure, I opened the printer glass, took out the white photographic paper, and placed it carefully into the developing fluid, at exactly 68 degrees Fahrenheit, in the plastic tray and started the stopwatch. Using the tongs, I turned the paper upside down and excitedly watched as an image magically appeared in the red light, becoming progressively darker every few seconds. At exactly sixty seconds, I transferred the picture to the "stop-bath" tray next for thirty seconds, washing off the developing fluid, and then placed it in the next tray with the fixing solution for sixty seconds, rinsed it in water, and turned on the room light. The portrait was way too dark, and it didn't look anything like the same picture that was professionally printed by the drug store. There was an image, something visible where minutes before there had been only an invisible image on a blank white piece of paper.

"It looks terrible."

"What did we do wrong?"

"I don't know. Let's try it again with a fresh piece of photographic paper."

"Okay. Maybe if we use less light it will be better."

Once more we repeated the process of placing the photographic paper and the negative into the contact printer.

This time I exposed the photographic paper for ten seconds before turning off the light, ten seconds less than the first attempt.

When I turned on the light after putting the paper through the developer, rinse, and fixer, the picture was too light, with facial features not contrasted enough to be able to see them well.

"This is terrible. I didn't think it was going to be this hard."

"Let's just do it again."

"You remember that story Mister Lamont told us about how gunners in the First World War worked out how to aim their mortars at the enemy?"

"Yeah. So?"

"They looked through binoculars to see how far the enemy was and made a calculation about the angle of the mortar and then fired. They looked at where the explosive landed. If it landed behind the enemy, they changed the angle and fired again. If it landed in front of the enemy, they fired a third shot starting with an angle between the two that they had already used. That would be the one that hit the target. We have to do that with our next attempt."

"Hey, dummy, we're not firing mortars."

"You're such an idiot. I know we're not firing mortars. But it is the same idea, don't you see?"

"Maybe. Instead of exposing the photographic paper to ten or twenty seconds, we're going to do fifteen seconds."

"Exactly."

Twenty years later, I used similar logic while doing lab research at UCLA.

That time, it worked perfectly. We were so excited, we carried the developed wet photograph out into the garden to show Moses, the gardener, who smiled and spoke to us in Sotho, which neither of us could understand. In my adult life in the lab, the experiences of trial and error in my childhood photographic lab reminded me how to keep going when experiments didn't work out perfectly, trying out different combinations or variables, creating new ideas.

We printed more pictures from the old negatives. Some came out well, and it was difficult to do perfectly every time because there were many aspects that could vary. By trial and error, trying different negatives, developers, and temperatures, we learned how to vary light and dark contrasts and how to focus our attention to which part of a picture we wanted to highlight. After spending a lot of time and many pieces of expensive photographic paper on getting the exactly perfect print, I found a perfect answer in the photography book.

"Hey, I've got an idea. If we expose the whole piece of paper for ten seconds, and then we cover strips with cardboard, we can use only one piece of paper to tell us whether ten, fifteen, or twenty seconds is the best."

"What are you talking about?"

"I'll show you."

I took the contact printer with a fresh piece of photographic paper and turned on the light for ten seconds. Then I covered three quarters of the paper with cardboard, leaving only one quarter exposed for a further three seconds. I moved the cardboard so only half of the paper was covered. Now I knew that the first quarter would have been exposed to sixteen seconds, and the next quarter to thirteen seconds. I repeated this with three quarters exposed for a further three seconds and then with the whole photograph exposed for another three seconds. The developed print had four different exposure times, and I chose the one that seemed best. Some pictures looked best with thirteen seconds, some with sixteen. We had worked out a way to save photographic paper because we only used two pieces per negative as opposed to three or more. The simple commonsense approach to solving problems by reading "how to" books or published papers or speaking to experts who had already done the procedure saved me countless hours of work and experimental time in my career.

Seeing how well I did with taking pictures and developing them, my parents gave me a Rolleiflex Twin Lens Reflex camera that took square two-and-a-quarter inch pictures for my tenth birthday. This was a major step up in quality for me, and now I could see better views in the view finder than I had with my box camera, vary the lens opening, also known as the *f*-stop, and the speed of the shutter. My box camera had no options for *f*-stop or shutter speed.

My Rollei pictures kept improving, and I experimented with varying the *f*-stop and the shutter speeds. I also learned to pick different films, learning that some film was deliberately made to be more sensitive than others. If I was taking pictures where the light was low, like indoors, I used a faster film, and if I was outdoors in brilliant sunshine, I used a slower film. These experiences proved invaluable in my scientific career later.

The Rollei had focusing knobs on the side. The Kodak box camera could not be focused. It had a fixed *f*-stop which was designed to keep most objects in focus. I soon discovered the concept of "depth of field," the distance between the nearest and the farthest objects that are in acceptably sharp focus in an image. Without understanding the physics and mathematics of light and lenses, I came to understand the marks on the focusing dial of the camera that showed me how near the nearest and furthest object in each photograph were in focus. All of this became even more clear to me some years later, including the mathematical formulas that I mastered when I took physics in high school.

My developing and printing skills continued to improve, and since Colin had lost interest, I did photography with Melvyn, a school friend who lived a block away. He also had a Rolleiflex camera, and we developed black and white film in plastic film tanks, bought our chemicals together in bulk, compared pictures, shared our growing expertise, and, after doing contact printing for four years, built an enlarger together at age fourteen since buying one in the store was too expensive.

By carefully examining enlargers in the photographic store and studying books, we created an apparatus from an incandescent light bulb, a cheap condensing lens, a film holder for the negative and the lens of my father's folding camera for projection. When the camera was fully unfolded it provided the correct focus distance from the film. By opening the back of the camera, we could place the film holder with a negative in the exact plane where the film would normally be when the folding camera was used for taking pictures. We converted the large walk-in cupboard in my bedroom into a darkroom. We were ready to try it out.

Our first focused image, achieved by adjusting the length of a light-tight bellows of the folding camera, projected onto the baseboard. The 8 x 10-inch photographic paper in a holder on the base board of our crude, homemade contraption received the projected image. Time flowed as we excitedly did the test strip to get the best picture contrast. We felt like explorers setting off on an expedition into unknown parts. Edmund Hillary had recently scaled mount Everest, and we knew how triumphant he must have felt standing on the top of the highest mountain for the first time. We held our breaths as we turned on the lights and watched as the image focused on the photographic paper.

Our excitement mounted as my father's enlarged portrait, taken a few weeks before with my Rollei, appeared in the developer. Having just read about Louis Pasteur and Robert Koch and their discoveries of micro-organisms at the end of the nineteenth century, understanding their triumphant feelings that proved their imagined ideas, picturing their excitement as they realized how their discoveries would change the world, dreaming of new experiments that they would do to further enhance their ideas, gave me an insight into how the process of discovery and problem solving are vital components of research endeavors and advances in every field of life. I went into the living room to show my parents the masterpiece I had just created, and they were astounded.

I had learned several lessons from my experiences developing and printing pictures, lessons that enhanced my future ability to do scientific experiments in my adult life, understand physics, using my hands to coordinate with my brain, and anticipating how my life in scientific research and surgical oncology might develop in the future.

Melvyn and I had discovered the power of looking within to identify our capacity to be curious and creative and to express ourselves by producing something that would create for us core identities, he as a musician and me as a clinical scientist.

Chapter 4

Hodgkin's Disease

Grandma Taube had survived anti-Semitism, the pogroms of Russia, and the Pale of Jewish Settlement, and, as a sixteen year-old, the harrowing journey in steerage on a Union Castle ship from England to South Africa with her poverty-stricken family, carrying her prized possession, a box of pictures of family graves in the Jewish cemetery in Zagare, north-eastern Lithuania, close to the Latvian border, and childhood memories, some happy, some terrifying, of a small town where half the population was Jewish.

She cooked old-fashioned recipes and drank Ceylon tea out of a glass while holding a cube of sugar between her teeth and filled my evenings with stories, told in a broken English with a heavy eastern European accent, of her family and her life in Lithuania and her experiences in her adopted country. There were stories of her early life, some filled with mystical superstitious overtones, from the old country. In her adopted country, living near Johannesburg, she had lots of tales about people of all types, interspersed with a little gossip about neighbors and family, including one of a friend who stole a loaf of bread in 1922, when times were tough, to how she had married my grandfather in 1905 in a double wedding with her brother Louis. Her favorite stories were always about her ancestors buried in Zagare, and she often took me into her bedroom where she pointed to the framed pictures of the graves, translating the Hebrew and Yiddish on the gravestones for me.

There had been lots of illness and tragedy, many "miscarriages," her personal bout of typhoid fever treated in the Johannesburg General Hospital in 1907, loss of her son, Abe, from "peritonitis" at age nineteen, a bout of peritonitis in my mother, her youngest child, at age sixteen, and many other devastatingly sad stories of epidemics, injuries, and deaths of family and friends. I was an avid listener, urging her to tell me more as I imagined what it must have been like to live in the "old days."

Grandma lived in Brakpan, forty miles from Johannesburg, in a one-bedroom cottage, built using the plans of a Scottish hunting lodge my grandfather bought from an advertisement in a popular magazine of the time, on a five-acre farm owned by his eldest son, my Uncle Nathan. She loved the cottage, as did I, with its quaint bedroom, dining room, sitting room, kitchen, pantry, and bathroom, filled with old framed photographs hanging on the walls, including her wedding picture, and a very old radio in one corner of the dining room, which crackled while it gave my grandfather the news of the world every night and old-fashioned music during the day.

My grandfather, Chaim, a surly, tough, sometimes harsh peasant from Memel in West Lithuania, who established a hardware store in Brakpan to support the exploding gold mining industry, died when I was eleven, and Grandma Taube, in her seventies, went on extended visits, in sequence, to her six remaining children. Once a year, she spent two months in our house in Johannesburg. Returning from school, I eagerly sat with her at the dining room table every afternoon, drank tea, and "schmoozed." These were cozy and intimate discussions where I quizzed her, encouraging her to gossip about her life and answer some of my more pressing questions about how to live a meaningful life. She always had an opinion, and despite my more advanced understanding of science, language, and modern life, I valued her wisdom.

Taube loved to listen to my stories about my friends, the teachers, and my curiosity. One day, after a flurry of questions, she laughed as she said: "You're such a *pochemuchka*."

"A what?"

"*Pochemuchka*."

"What's that?"

"Well, it's like you are a why-boy. You are a curious child, always asking many questions."

"Is that bad?"

"No, no, no! It is a good thing. But, you know, you have to be careful because sometimes people get a little uncomfortable with questions."

This comment was typical of grandma's "peasant wisdom." She had gained knowledge and understanding through observation. She had learned to "see" the cows on the farm while I could frequently look at the same cows and perhaps learn about their breed, diet, habits, origins, and many other details from reading books but without really "knowing" the cows. By seeing these animals, she gained a deep understanding of their nature, and she called them by friendly, made-up names. The animals "talked to her" about their fitness, health, and well-being every day through their hair coat, body condition, and manure. She sensed things in people in much the same way, discerning attitudes in others that I did not see. Her presence connected her to a space, an essence, even more apparent when she met other Lithuanian immigrants, the room filled with a warmth, togetherness, and familiarity. She exuded a freshness, a breeze around her, a friendliness that made me feel more alive. She poured love into me and other children, and when I was close to her, just the very kinship, the proximity gave me a sense of clarification. Her presence enhanced my understanding of life, love, compassion, beauty, and reality.

Fascinated by her observations, decisions, wisdom, and her survival skills I asked her a question one day: "Grandma, how do you understand so much?"

"This comes from years of looking."

"What do you mean by 'looking?'"

"Well, you should watch everyone passing by. And you should watch when they talk to you."

"I don't understand. I do look at people, but they don't always want me to look at them. Sometimes people yell at me and ask me what I'm staring at."

"Well, you must learn to look without them seeing that you're looking."

"How do you do that?"

"Just a quick look will do. Just with the eyes. Then look straight ahead."

"But what are you looking for, Grandma?"

"You have to learn yourself."

"But how do I start?"

"See exactly what is happening."

"Then what?"

"When somebody talks, listen to the face, the eyes, the arms, and the body."

"How do I do that? I don't understand."

"Listen to what I tell you. Up to now you have lived only with the words, right?"

"Yes, but that's the only way to hear what they're saying."

"Oy, you're being such a *schlemiel*."

"What does that mean?'

"It means you shouldn't be so simple minded."

"But I don't understand how you can listen to a face."

"Because the face talks. The eyes, they talk too. And the body talks."

"How can I hear those parts is what I want to know."

"A person may be saying 'I love you,' and his eyes may be denying it. Another person may be smiling with his lips, and his eyes may be scorning you. Someone else may be saying 'hello' and holding your hand, and his whole being may be criticizing you."

"Really? Are you telling me that words are deceptive?"

"Yes, that's it. Look for the true meaning of the words."

"When did you start doing that, Grandma?"

"It doesn't matter, my Dovidel. You're not too young. You should start sometime, and now is the time."

"Is there an easy way to do it?"

"There is no shortcut. Just do it every day. With practice, you will find out."

I learned a lot of facts at school, but I understood my grandma when she said: "Knowledge is very easy; knowing and understanding is very difficult." My task was to learn how to know and to combine that knowing with understanding.

Taube had six children and lots of grandchildren, and I knew that she loved them, but I believed she loved me more than anyone else. When somebody loves you, pretense is unnecessary. You can drop all your defenses. I could trust that she would not take advantage of me, and she would keep our secrets to herself. Being defenseless in her presence was soothing, and I could be myself and not play games, making me happy. I could go back to her if I was uncertain and admit that I felt that way, a feeling that I couldn't expose to my school friends and teachers. I could not even be that open with my parents.

A caring confidant, like Grandma, is someone who understands your past, believes in your future, and accepts you just the way you are.

Four years of "grandma's visits" passed, and although at age fifteen I was busy learning, reading, playing sports, discovering girls, and planning for my future, and even though it meant choosing her over my friends, I preferred talking to her just before family dinner.

One day when returning home from school, I was surprised to find the cars of all five of my mother's brothers parked in front of our house. Young teenage boys don't think too much about personal tragedies, even though they might be aware of those possibilities, and at first, I didn't think anything was wrong. I was curious to find out what everybody was doing there, in the middle of the week, and that my mother hadn't told me we would have visitors from out of town for dinner.

I breezily opened the front door, walked into the vestibule, and announced I was home. To my left, the door to the living room was closed, and I heard voices coming from that direction, and I opened it and started to walk in.

Grannie Taube was sitting in a comfortable armchair, and she smiled at me. My uncles John, Cecil, Louis, and Barney stood in a circle around Grandma. My mother, sitting on one of the sofas next to Uncle Nathan, looked strained and uncomfortable and she said: "David, we're having a private conversation, and we'd like you to leave us for a while."

"What's going on, Mom?"

"I'll tell you later."

The last time I had seen my mother look so disturbed was when my grandfather had died four years previously. Something about her facial expression told me something bad was happening. Taube had advised me to look deeply at the face, and now I had knowledge that I felt deep inside me somewhere, a "knowing" that started my internal dialogue. Someone was sick. Who could it be? Was it my mother? My father wasn't there. He was still at work. It likely wasn't one of my uncles. It must be Grandma. Otherwise, why would all her sons be there without their wives? What kind of sickness could it be?

I went to my room and tried to think about whether Grandma had looked sick. She hadn't complained or showed any signs of illness. She hadn't been in bed, where sick people often were. I was worried in a way that I had never been before. Her presence, her very being was vital to my happiness, and I began to think about her age, and to think about a condition so serious that she might not survive. My mind went to scenes from movies where death was depicted. Mario Lanza playing the Great Caruso came vividly back to me as I remembered how awful I felt with the dying scene. I was scared.

My mother found me and sat me down to tell me that Grannie had a lump in her neck and the surgeon did a biopsy.

"What's a biopsy?"

"He took out a lymph node, and the lab said it was Hodgkin's disease."

I immediately remembered the word lymph from the day I had visited the Johannesburg library and started reading a book on the lymphatic system.

"What does it mean? What's going to happen?"

"She will get radiation."

"How will she feel? Will it make her sick?"

"The doctor said she should be all right because it is only in her neck. The radiation might make her mouth a little dry, but she should be able to do it well. She'll be staying with us for an extra six weeks while she gets the treatment, and I want you to help her with anything she needs."

"Of course, Mom.'

"Go and speak to her. She wants to talk to you."

I felt strange as I walked towards the living room, knowing that my Taube had a disease that I had never heard of and didn't know anything about. I imagined she would be terrified of the diagnosis and reluctant to get radiation treatment.

"Hi, Grandma."

"Nu, so how are you, Dovidel?"

"I'm well."

She looked deeply into my eyes, and I felt that she was able to see right through to the back of my brain. Usually when she did that, I had no secrets, and I talked openly and honestly, never trying to hide anything. She had to know that I felt awkward.

"Don't worry about me. I'll be fine."

She looked fine. I noticed a little white bandage above her collar bone on the left side of her neck.

"Does it hurt?"

"No, not at all."

"Mom told me about the treatment. When will they start?"

"Next week. Don't worry about me. I'll be fine. We'll have our little talks just like before."

"Okay.'

The next day, at the Johannesburg library, I asked the librarian if she could help me find a book on Hodgkin's disease.

"You may have to go to a medical library."

"I know there's a book somewhere here on the lymphatic system that I looked at four years ago. I can't remember where it is. Maybe that would be a good way to start."

She found the book, and I took it to one of the library tables and started to read about the lymphatic system, this time with a great deal of intention, concentrating intently on learning more about lymph nodes and the lymphatic system.

My interrogation of lymph, lymphatics, lymph nodes, and the lymphatic system had begun in earnest, preparing my mind for future discovery and understanding.

Chapter 5

Splenomegaly

During my internal medicine rotation as a fourth-year medical student at Coronation Hospital, the main public hospital for mixed-race people of the Johannesburg area, I was assigned to do the admission history and physical examination of Derek, a Cape Colored man in his late forties who was anemic and had an enlarged spleen.

I had already done learning rotations in various specialties at the Johannesburg General Hospital, for white patients only, and Baragwanath Hospital, reserved for Black African patients only. Coronation Hospital, a general hospital opened in 1944 in the suburb of Coronationville, a township for colored people during the South African apartheid era of government-mandated separation of racial groups, was one of the academic hospitals of my medical school.

Sitting on a chair next to my new patient's bed, note pad and pen at the ready, I took a detailed history, including his current symptoms, his past illnesses, surgical procedures, his medications, his habits, and his origins. The Afrikaans word, *bruinmense*, for this multiracial man was quite literally "brown persons." "Coloreds" were a distinct population of people whose ancestors were a combination of ethnicities, an ancestry from more than one of the various Southern African populations, including whites from Europe, Khoisan, Bantu, Afrikaner, Austronesian, East Asian, or South Asian. Since his papers sub-classified him as "Cape Colored," I assumed he was a mixture of one of the various ethnic populations of the Cape, the southwest portion of South Africa, and Malays, a population that had been brought as slaves by the Dutch East India Company in the seventeenth, eighteenth, and nineteenth centuries to the Cape of Good Hope from the Malay archipelago and Dutch Malacca. Many Malay slaves had children with African partners.

Derek, with a toothless smile, was quite jovial and friendly while I examined him from the top of his head to the bottom of his feet. I carefully noted all the physical features, paying attention to his pallor, a sign of anemia, and his enlarged spleen, which I could easily feel while he took in a deep breath, and I placed my right hand in the left upper part of his abdomen.

"Hey, Doc, what do think? Why am I so tired?"

"Well, Derek, you are anemic, and that's enough to create a strain on your heart and make you feel tired."

"How come I'm like that?"

"I tell you what—I have to discuss your case with my chief and see what he says. We have to do a few tests, and then you and I can talk some more."

"Okay."

Upon discussion with the intern on the case, we ordered blood tests and some X-rays. The next day we had a result that seemed to explain his anemia. He had sickle cell disease, a disease of black Africans that causes severe anemia and requires blood transfusions, amongst other treatments. I presented his case to the team on "teaching rounds" that afternoon. The discussion from the main attending internist and the chief registrar and a few of the "house staff" centered around the diagnosis, epidemiology, genetics, and biology of hemoglobin S, or HbS, a structurally abnormal hemoglobin with one amino acid changed from the usual adult hemoglobin. I had quickly read about sickle cell disease in the textbook before rounds, and I was surprised that none of my teachers had any doubt about the diagnosis. The sickle cell test on whole blood had shown the typical appearance of the abnormal red blood cells, converted from the usual oval cells to a rigid sickle-like shape. That was enough for my team, but I noticed some incongruous features that didn't fit the diagnosis. I felt anxious in the presence of these more experienced clinicians, since I was just a medical student, to challenge the undisputed diagnosis, but since my photographic experiences, I had learned to observe in a certain way and to find connections and deeper meanings. My heart beating fast, my mouth dry, I stammered a little as I asked: "Is it usual for a patient with sickle-cell anemia to have splenomegaly?"

The chief looked erudite and completely comfortable when he said: "Ten percent of patients with this disease have a splenomegaly."

He had put me in my place, dismissing my question completely. I did not know enough about the disease to challenge him further, but I studied it deeply over the next day and used the reasoning I had gleaned from reading *Sherlock Holmes* mysteries to develop my case. The renowned fictional detective relied on detailed observation and "connecting the dots," an astute way of collecting, analyzing, and linking the clues from detective cases.

Patients with sickle cell disease have severe health problems starting in early childhood, anemia, swelling of the hands and feet, repeated bacterial infections, various types of acute crises of various organs, and chronic pain, none of which had occurred in my patient, which he confirmed when I went back and asked him directly.

The presence of an enlarged spleen—splenomegaly—bothered me the most. The first patient diagnosed with sickle cell anemia in the United States, in the nineteenth century, a run-away slave, was executed, and an autopsy revealed he had no spleen. In many patients with the disease, episodes of inadequate blood flow, caused by sickle-shaped red blood cells that obstruct capillaries and restrict blood flow to an organ, result in acute pain and death of tissue; the spleen, often bearing the brunt of these tissue-destroying episodes, is often destroyed before the end of childhood. When tissues die in the body, the dead tissue is often removed by so-called phagocytic cells, resulting in what appears to be a complete absence of the organ. Yet, incongruously, our patient had an enlarged spleen.

Before I went back to the chief, I explored another question in the library: does sickle cell disease occur in any other ethnic groups outside of Black Africans? Could a man of his ethnic origin have sickle cell disease?

I discovered that a person with sickle cell disease inherits two abnormal copies of the beta globin gene that makes hemoglobin, one from each parent.

The disease occurs in black people of African origin. To have both genes, both of the patient's parents would either have the disease or both would need to have had one gene inherited from a black ancestor. A person with a single abnormal gene copy does not usually have symptoms and is said to have sickle cell trait, a carrier of the abnormal gene in one chromosome but not the other. Carriers have symptoms only if they are deprived of oxygen (for example, while climbing a mountain) or while severely dehydrated. My patient was not pure black, so he might possibly have inherited one abnormal globin allele from a black ancestor, making him a carrier. The so-called sickle cell trait does not produce anemia or splenomegaly. Therefore, his anemia could not have been due to sickle cell disease.

Excited by my detective work, filled with moments of pure joy when my challenge to the "obvious" diagnosis confirmed my doubts about the true diagnosis, a joy that I had previously experienced when delving into the deeper meanings of stories in my high school English literature classes and my discoveries in my photographic lab, I wanted to share my excitement with the chief.

He was in his office when I asked if I could discuss the case with him, and I revealed my research and discoveries. Fortunately, to my relief, he was interested. He could have treated me as an obnoxious, precocious medical student and dismissed my observations, but instead, he complimented me on my persistence and the logical way I had delved more deeply into the subject.

"Your observations are pertinent. Now, we have a problem because we don't know what caused his anemia. Did you think about that?" he asked.

"Yes, I investigated all the other common causes of anemia because I thought even with asymptomatic sickle cell trait, he could still get one of the other common forms of anemia."

"What did you find?"

"His blood smear shows hypochromic, microcytic red cells with anisocytosis and poikilocytosis, and the mean corpuscular volume is low."

"What's the usual cause of that type of anemia?"

"Iron deficiency."

"How do you identify that as a cause?"

"We tested his blood and his iron levels; iron binding capacity and ferritin levels are normal, which excludes the diagnosis of iron deficiency anemia."

"What other anemias can be microcytic and hypochromic?"

"Thalassemia and sideroblastic anemia."

"Does this patient have sideroblasts in his blood?"

"No."

"Does he have thalassemia?"

"I don't know. I think we have to do hemoglobin electrophoresis to help us make that diagnosis."

"We don't see thalassemia in our patient population, and I've never had to order that test. I'm not sure if the lab does hemoglobin electrophoresis to detect different types of hemoglobin. We need to find out."

It didn't take long to find out from Professor Stein in the Clinical Pathology laboratory at the Johannesburg General Hospital that rare inherited disorders of red blood cells, called hemoglobinopathies, were so uncommon that they didn't offer the electrophoresis test.

Remembering how I had made a photographic enlarger from very cheap components, cobbled together to produce a picture, I asked the professor whether I could use his lab to do hemoglobin electrophoresis to help confirm the diagnosis of thalassemia trait combined with sickle cell trait. The internal medicine team at Coronation Hospital thought that we could tentatively settle on the clinical diagnosis of sickle cell thalassemia, and they endorsed the idea of me doing electrophoresis on the patient's blood.

Stein was not exactly enthusiastic.

"You might learn how to do the electrophoresis, and it would show you Hb S migrating separately from Hb A. Hb S is not found in normal human blood, and its presence would confirm what we already know; the patient has sickle cell hemoglobin in his blood. The migration patterns of hemoglobin in patients with thalassemia will not show an abnormal band of hemoglobin, so you cannot easily diagnose the thalassemia trait that you think might exist in this patient."

For a moment, I felt confused, uncertain as to how I would proceed. But there had to be a way.

"How does hemoglobin electrophoresis help make the diagnosis of thalassemia?" I asked.

"By finding an increase in hemoglobin A_2, Hb A_2, which is normally present in low amounts in normal human blood. Hb A_2 may be increased in beta thalassemia or in people who are heterozygous for the beta thalassemia gene, like in your patient."

"Is Hb A_2 elevated in patients with sickle cell trait?"

"No, it is not."

"So, all I have to do is learn how to do cellulose acetate gel electrophoresis."

I told Stein of my many years of developing and printing black and white film at home and how I had made my own enlarger.

"That sounds good. You may already have some skills that will help. I'll ask Doctor Basil Bradlow and his laboratory technicians to facilitate your progress. The equipment and supplies to do the electrophoresis are available for you to use. After you extract hemoglobin from the red blood cells and do a cellulose acetate electrophoresis on the solution, work with Bradlow. You will need to play around with temperatures, times, the amount of current, the composition of the buffer, and many other variables."

Ruth, the technician assigned to help me, had enough to do in her daily lab duties, and she was quite irritated with me trying to do the assay. I quickly discovered that something as simple as getting a pure solution of hemoglobin was not all that easy.

Eventually, after a few weeks of trial and error and a few dozen attempts, I had the technique that produced a perfect cellulose acetate gel hemoglobin electrophoresis. I shared it with Doctor Bradlow who looked at it carefully and pointed to the lines that represented Hb A, Hb A_2, and fetal hemoglobin, Hb F. Since the specimen was from a normal volunteer, the Hb A_2 and Hb F electrophoresis bands were very faint.

"Next, we need to try the hemoglobin from your patient."

Before starting my project, I had taken five tubes of blood from the patient, made hemoglobin preparations, and placed them in the freezer. I produced a great migration pattern from a thawed aliquot of the patient's hemoglobin, which showed the Hb S. The Hb A_2 and Hb F strips seemed a little more prominent than in the normal control hemoglobin, and unskilled at how quantitative analysis in the lab needed more than just a casual observation, I jumped for joy, elated beyond belief that I had proved the diagnosis in my patient.

Bradlow, however, was unimpressed.

"That's inadequate," he said. "It's a start but not proof. You need to establish a normal range for Hb A_2, Hb A, and Hb F in at least twenty normal people by measuring the percentages of those proteins. Ruth can show you how to scan those strips and get a range of normal for Hb A, Hb A_2 and Hb F. Go and do that and then come back to me."

It dawned on me that clinical conclusions and laboratory conclusions were in two different spheres. Laboratory scientists were trained to do repeated experiments, to make sure of their conclusions before they reported the result. Clinicians put a lot of clinical information together, developed a list of possible diagnoses, and eventually excluded all but one or two. The final clinical diagnosis was not always exact. Initially frustrated by the slow, meticulous approach to determining the percentages of three different hemoglobins in blood from normal people, I managed to calm my impatient brain down into the rhythm required to produce accurate, repeatable lab results. Constructing tables, I wrote the numbers down for each normal control, and after a few weeks, I reported to Bradlow that the average Hb A was 96 percent, Hb A_2 1.5 to 3 percent and Hb F about 1 percent.

"That's good. Now it's time to test your patient's hemoglobin. Remember to run a strip that contains normal hemoglobin at the same time. Repeat it twice to make sure you have a good result that can be confidently reported to your chief."

Remembering the excitement that I felt with my first printed photograph in my makeshift dark room at home twelve years previously, I impatiently measured my patient's hemoglobins.

There is no accurate way to describe the feeling when one completes an experiment, and the result is so confirming that one is ready to yell "eureka," like Archimedes in Ancient Greece, an elation that may also have overtaken Einstein when he discovered relativity, Newton when the apple hit his head and he realized the importance of gravity, or the California miners finding a gold nugget. When one is elated, you aren't just happy; you're over-the-moon excited, bursting with an irrepressible pride, and I had to tell Bradlow immediately. Even though it was dark outside, well after dinner time, and even hesitating one moment while thinking it might be impolite to call him then, I could not wait until morning.

"Sir, I have the results of my electrophoresis runs on Derek's hemoglobin," I announced breathlessly. "His Hb A_2 is three times higher than normal, and his Hb F is twice normal."

"Good. I'll be happy to look at it tomorrow to check your calculations."

Disappointed that he didn't seem to be jumping for joy, I waited for his confirmation the next day. I was triumphant when he said: "It looks like you have proven this patient has sickle cell thalassemia."

I smiled as he examined my workbook, untidy and crammed with comments, accumulated over four weeks of experiments.

"I'm not sure how we can explain the epidemiology of this rare finding," he said.

"I've been thinking about that a lot. Thalassemia is most commonly found in populations scattered around the Mediterranean Sea, and sickle cell disease is most commonly found in Africa. I'd like to do a study of Derek's family which might help determine how he inherited the disease."

Bradlow looked carefully at me and expressed a combination of interest and caution.

"If you're really interested in doing this study, you should construct a family tree and work out how many members from both sides of the family you can find and how interested they might be in donating blood. Ask Doctor Dunn to help you. Once you have that information, come back to me, and we can work out how much time and supplies we might need."

Impatient to get this all done, I soon found the hurdles and roadblocks almost insurmountable. The first hurdle was getting permission to visit Derek at home in Coronationville. In apartheid South Africa in 1964, it was difficult to convince the police that I wanted to visit a patient in a Colored Township for research purposes. The country was embroiled in the Rivonia treason trial involving Nelson Mandela and twelve co-defendants and racial violence was on the minds of many. Any white man who wanted to visit a colored man in his home might be plotting something dreadful. Finally, the police agreed to grant me a permit for one day. It was easier to convince my medical school professors once I summarized my research objectives.

Derek, feeling less tired after his blood transfusions in the hospital, invited his siblings, cousins, aunties, uncles, and as many of the children who could be there to a "big party." I created an abstracting sheet for each person aimed at documenting and creating a genetic tree. Armed with syringes, needles, Band-Aids, cotton, alcohol, and blood tubes in a large suitcase, enough for about one hundred people, I parked my car in the street outside his house early on a sunny and cloudless Sunday morning, and my medical school friend Roger and I were greeted at the front door. The grubby neighborhood showed signs of wear and poverty; discarded old newspapers, beer cans, and other garbage littered haphazard in the dusty streets and the poorly constructed sidewalks, and even in the front gardens of the brick homes. Shoeless boys in ragged clothes, yelling out names and laughing a lot, dribbled a homemade soccer ball past opponents, aiming at makeshift goals. Occasionally, a family in their Sunday-best walked by as they headed to the local church. A few of the houses had old, wrecked cars on the front lawns, where flower gardens were sparse.

The inside of the house was already filled with dozens of people, some drinking homemade wine and beer, and Derek introduced us. I found a small wooden table in one of the rooms and carefully arranged my supplies while telling everyone how grateful I was that they had agreed to meet, give us some information, and have their blood drawn. I told them why we were so interested in finding out whether they had something in their blood that would help me identify Derek's origins and to determine how he had inherited a very rare type of blood disease.

Roger and I spent the whole day drawing blood, accurately labelling the tubes and completing the abstracting forms I had created. The blood drawing was tedious but much easier than obtaining the personal information, a nightmare to accomplish, taking a lot longer than I had anticipated. None of the people we interrogated were sure of their origins, and in the end, we had to accept simple demographic data about age, sex, place of birth, and how they were related to Derek. Some were not related in any way, but they thought it would be a good idea to volunteer, which seemed strange until I realized that everyone thought they were being paid for their contribution; I told them I was a medical student and had no money to share except the twenty rand in my pocket, which I gave to Derek.

Although many of the people worked in factories and businesses owned by white bosses, they had not seen white people in their homes in the township.

Neighbors wanted to see this event, and the crowd was raucous and became louder with more cheap wine and beer drunk. Derek's wife, a colored woman with no Cape Malay or Cape Colored ancestors, and some of her friends served food that had originated in the Malay community of the Cape of Good Hope. Cape Malay samoosas, triangular, spicy, meat-filled pastries, were so spicy they brought tears to my eyes. I also tried the bredie, a mutton stew; bobotie, spiced minced meat baked with an egg-based topping; sosaties, meat cooked on skewers; and koeksisters, fried dough infused in syrup or honey. They tasted different to those same dishes that I had eaten at home, probably because they were cooked in the traditional Malay fashion with original recipes possibly centuries old.

The medical histories of our blood donors were often long, the folks all anxious to talk endlessly about themselves and their lives to two guys in white coats. We focused on direct questions regarding symptoms or past histories suggestive of thalassemia or sickle cell disease which none had. They all had questions about treatment for many unrelated minor ailments that bothered them, taking advantage of the presence of the young "doctors."

Our blood drawing party continued into the late afternoon, interspersed with more laughter, alcohol, food, and Cape Malay folk songs of Dutch origin, and we left, exhausted but happy that we had accomplished our task. After a brief compulsory stop at the local police station to report our completed mission, we took all the samples back to the Johannesburg General Hospital and placed the tubes in the fridge, ready for processing the next day.

Interspersed with medical school lectures, I processed all the samples over the next few weeks, measuring Hb A_2 and Hb F percentages and finding the occasional sample with Hb S, enough for me to analyze and interpret the likely origins of the sickle cell and thalassemia genes.

The library research I did to help me further understand sickle cell thalassemia and how it was present in a Cape Malay man was somewhat like the library research I had done in high school and medical school. I discovered that Malays were often skilled fishermen, farmers, furniture makers, dressmakers, and coopers, and Derek was a manager in the textile industry. His wife, like many colored women, was a service worker in the food industry. I also discovered that thalassemia was most common in people of Italian, Greek,

Middle Eastern, South Asian, and African descent. I could not tell exactly where Derek inherited his thalassemia genes, but the sickle cell gene was most likely from a Bantu male or a Khoisan female. Neither his mother nor his father were alive, and I didn't have enough specimens from their generation to be able to tell which of the disease genes came from his mother's side and which from his father.

Bradlow was very supportive of the whole effort I had put into this study and suggested that we submit a complete paper to the South African Medical Journal. He also suggested we submit the paper to the Association of Medical Students of South Africa (AMSSA) for their annual meeting in Cape Town in 1965.

I presented the paper to the AMSSA conference, my first time standing in front of a large national audience, and after showing pictures of the electrophoresis strips, the sickle cells in the peripheral blood, demographic data of the family who donated blood, tables showing the percentages of Hb A_2 and Hb F in the entire group, and describing the history of the Cape Malays, I was awarded first prize in the competition. The South African Medical Journal published my paper entitled: "Sickle-cell thalassemia in Johannesburg; A case study and family study" in 1968.

Professor Stein's Clinical Pathology Department gave each student an assignment to complete a major review of a subject, and I chose "The molecular basis of the hemoglobinopathies." I had a few months to complete this project, and it dovetailed well with my sickle cell thalassemia project and with my prior experience learning photography.

1964 was a particularly exciting time for me as a medical student studying well-established biological, biochemical, and physiological systems in the animal body to discover another world in cutting-edge science, namely, the new molecular biology of cells. My professors were aware of the revolution that had been initiated by the discovery of the structure of DNA in 1953, but it was still not clearly understood how genes produced proteins in cells. Many such proteins had important functions, as was clear from my study of sickle cell thalassemia. I focused my report on how "one gene could produce one protein," in my case, Hb S. I discovered the production of proteins by cells was accomplished through the processes of transcription, via messenger RNA, and translation, or ribosomal reading of the sequence of mRNA bases, information that modern-day high-school sophomores know, but which fifty-five years ago we weren't even taught in medical school. My reading took me on a wild ride through papers in top class journals, bringing me into contact with the work of Jacob and Monod, recipients of the 1965 Nobel Prize in Medicine, which I read repeatedly with limited understanding, but which allowed me to write a paper that received the second highest grade in the class, and was published in *The Leech* in 1965.

The experience of creating a hypothesis, designing an experiment, doing the research, making and recording observations, thinking about the results, doing the critical analysis, writing the details, carefully and repeatedly editing the entire experience, and adding one more brick to the wall of knowledge confirmed for me a belief which I adopted for my career in science and medicine. I had complete faith in Enlightenment scientific methods. Nothing seemed more satisfying than questioning the established "truths" of the time and to find new truths.

By exposing a clinical diagnosis that seemed flawed, I had embraced an objective, value-free, scientific worldview, free of myth and religious fervor, to guide me in determining what was true. Each page of every textbook contained multiple dogmatic statements, some based on instincts and faith without scientific proof, and I began to look for these "mistakes" and to believe that I could easily find ways to investigate and challenge unscientific dogma.

Curiosity and hard work were ahead of me.

Chapter 6

Lymphadenopathy

The mysterious world of diseases, a world filled with conditions affecting organs, body systems, cells, and tissues, meant plowing through enormously thick textbooks, memorizing thousands of new words and concepts and thousands more ideas related to causes, or pathogenesis, of these mysterious conditions, almost all of them ending in "-itis," "-osis," "necrosis," or "failure," or starting with "ischemic," or "cancer of," or "obstruction of," or "calcification of," and some other choice words that penetrated my mind day and night for my entire third year of medical school.

My brain rebelled at this process, and I felt like a goose fattened by force-feeding corn with a feeding tube to make *pate de foie gras* from the over-fattened liver. Either I was too slow, needing extra time to understand and work through one new concept before being bombarded too quickly by another important pathogenetic mechanism, or I needed to think about the fascinating origins of those diseases and the people who discovered them. I wanted to hear the stories of the pioneers, digest them a little, imagine what it was like to see a disease that no one had previously seen, and get a sense of what those geniuses felt when they knew that they had found something new. While we were encouraged to explore those stories a little, acknowledging that many were first observed and reported at a remote time, we had to move on very quickly to the modern understanding of the disease and spend our time mastering that information.

The pathology department, was manned by serious-minded, dull, mostly old professors, whose somnolent lectures on all the diseases of Man were infused with blackboard diagrams, gross-looking photographs, or fixed specimens of diseased organs in well-marked glass containers, and who led us through smelly morning autopsies in the mortuary of the Johannesburg General Hospital.

Immediately following the early morning lecture, we walked across the street from the medical school on Hospital Hill to an old building, separate from the hospital, and which housed an old-fashioned lecture theater with hard wooden benches overlooking two marble tables, each supporting a new cadaver, dead human bodies used by the pathologists to identify disease sites and determine causes of death. Only those of us registered as medical students could enter this morbid space and Mister Momson, the bald, pudgy, toothless, morgue supervisor wearing a blood-stained apron and knee-high rubber boots, saw to it that we sat in alphabetic order for two hours, three days a week. He read out the names and checked them off as we entered the hallowed space. He had been hired some years before when, as a house painter, his first job in his youth, and while painting the outside of the morgue, he was fascinated with the cadavers inside and almost fell off his ladder one day while peering through the window into the inner sanctuary. This incident came to the attention of the pathologists who needed an assistant, and Momson was hired.

I'm surprised to this day that we, as young mischievous-minded students, never called him "Morbid Momson," for he certainly took his job seriously, making particularly sure that no student of color, in the apartheid era of South Africa, was admitted on days where there was a white cadaver. He obviously felt responsible for upholding the ridiculous belief that dark-skinned students should not be allowed to see autopsies on white people. He was responsible for identifying two students per day, in strict order, to don protective gowns, gloves, and shoe covers to assist the pathologist performing the autopsy.

When my turn came to assist, I had to suppress my natural instincts to be nauseated by the smell and the difficult feelings that welled up in me because of my fear of new corpses. I had already spent an entire year dissecting a cadaver in the anatomy department with no such fear, but the fresh bodies were different. They were recently dead and looked like people, filled with human colors, including yellow fat, the brain white and grey and recently the engine of the mind, alive-looking organs, like the liver, filled with red and bluish blood, and the entire body covered by skin that felt and looked like human skin, whereas my cadaver in the anatomy lab, pickled with preservative, the tissues drained of blood, looking un-human, the eye sockets empty looking because the eyes lost their turgor when preserved for months or years, the brain removed because it could not be adequately preserved inside the skull, and the skin feeling like cardboard, was different. The freshly dead person looked almost like he would open his eyes and look directly at me and say something. The eerie feeling was enhanced by Doctor Abrams, a young and vibrant pathologist, the only pathologist who had not yet taken on the grey, wan appearance of the cadavers they dissected, seemed especially interested in asking me a lot of questions, this heightened attention possible owing to the fact that he had met me socially because he was dating my cousin Phyllis.

"Describe the external appearance of the patient, Nathanson," said Abrams.

I felt as if my face was burning since I was in front of my classmates, and I was unsure of myself. I quickly took in a deep breath, imagined the format of the presentation that I had observed and studied previously and, using my best powers of observation, said: "Caucasian female, approximately thirty-five years old, about five feet, five inches tall, with a fresh vertical scar in her abdomen, intact teeth, multiple bruises on both arms, a rash on her left breast, and evidence of lividity."

Abrams was responsible for producing a complete report, and he quickly repeated what I had just said into a recording microphone present to one side of the marble slab bearing the body.

"What do you think the rash is?" he asked.

"I don't know."

"Describe the rash so your classmates at the back can help us."

"Well, it looks like little red flat macules in some of the lesions, and some project as small, fluid-filled blisters."

"Why is the rash confined to one side of the body?"

"I don't know."

He looked at the class, and someone said: "Could that be shingles?"

"Yes, that is indeed what this patient had according to the clinical notes. Why should a young woman like this have shingles?" He looked directly at me.

"I don't know."

"Do you know what causes shingles?"

"I think it's caused by reactivation of the varicella zoster virus, the same virus that causes chickenpox."

"What sorts of people get it?"

"I believe older people mainly."

"What is it about older people makes them more likely to get the disease?"

"I don't know.'

He looked up at the class. "Anybody?"

"Maybe it has something to do with the immune system and how it deteriorates with age."

"That is certainly likely," said Abrams.

He looked at the body and pointed to her neck.

"Did you notice the small scar in the lower left neck?"

I looked carefully, and there it was, just above the clavicle.

Even before he spoke again, I remembered my grandmother who had a lymph node in her neck biopsied and was treated for Hodgkin's disease with radiation.

According to her clinical notes, this patient went to her doctor complaining of a lump in her neck and was diagnosed with "lymphadenopathy." She had been referred to a surgeon who excised the enlarged lymph node and sent it to the lab. It was nodular sclerosing Hodgkin's disease, the same diagnosis that my grandmother had. Now it made more sense that she had shingles, since patients with lymphoid malignancies, like Hodgkin's disease, are at significantly higher risk of getting shingles.

The mind of a medical student studying all the diseases of Man is sometimes subject to bouts of hypochondria, an almost daily fear of either already having the disease being studied or of developing it in the future. I had noticed a lump on the left side of my own neck and had begun worrying that it could be something serious. Now here I was, with the body of a relatively young woman who had died of the disease. My mind worked overtime as I was convinced I, too, had the disease, and I would soon end up on a marble slab.

As we did the rest of the autopsy, examining all the organs after they were removed and dissected, with Abrams periodically dictating into the microphone to record the details, the cause of death was a large pulmonary embolus, a blood clot blocking blood flow to her lungs, which had developed eight days after a staging laparotomy operation, including removing her spleen, biopsy of her liver, excision of lymph nodes from various parts of the abdomen, and moving her ovaries to the middle of her pelvis next to her uterus to protect them from possible future radiation to that area. She had not died of Hodgkin's disease but of a surgical complication.

For days after that autopsy experience, I kept feeling the enlarged lymph node in my neck. I was convinced it was Hodgkin's disease. I asked one of my friends to examine my neck.

"You should probably see a surgeon," he said.

"Who should I see?"

"If it were me, I would go straight to the top. To the head of the surgery department, Professor DuPlessis."

I made an appointment, and so nervous that I was sweating, breathing rapidly and had a rapid pulse, I sat in the waiting room outside his office. His presence around the medical school was legendary, and I was terrified that he would tell me that I needed to have the node removed. After what seemed like many eons, his secretary told me to enter his office.

Sitting at his desk, the tall man with steely blue eyes, narrow lips, and broad shoulders that I would come to know well years later, wearing an impeccably clean white coat, asked me a few questions and examined my neck.

"My children have bigger lymph nodes than that. You probably had tonsillitis as a child and developed enlarged lymph nodes. Everyone gets those. Sometimes they stay around for many years and don't cause problems. You do not need to have them removed."

That was it. I was relieved, and I went back to study the immune system and lymph nodes, convinced that my repeated interaction with the lymphatic system, and my discovery that it was as mysterious as it had been a generation before, with little new discovered, that I should think about studying it more, so I could discover something unique.

Chapter 7

Anatomy

Professor Phillip Tobias, head of the anatomy department at Wits medical school, the proverbial *wunderkind* whose legendary, eloquent lectures resonated in my imagination from my time learning anatomy as a medical student, welcomed me back as a "table doc" thirteen months after graduating medical school in 1966 and immediately following my year as an intern managing patients in the hospital.

The position of table doctor was filled by six young doctors who wanted to train in one of the South African training programs in general surgery. The privilege of training in general surgery was dependent upon passing the primary examination of the fellowship of the South African College of Surgeons, requiring post-graduate written and oral examination in anatomy, physiology, and pathology. Only those who passed the examination could hope to gain a position in training programs in surgery. We all knew the pass rate for the primary examination was less than 20 percent. Most people who took the examination failed anatomy. The level of anatomic knowledge required of surgical trainees was very high, and although one could restudy from anatomy books and atlases, with memories of our days as second-year medical students spent dissecting a cadaver, it was generally understood that only those who had spent a year teaching anatomy to medical, dental, physical therapy, and occupational therapy students would pass the exam.

The six new table docs were introduced to the staff, a group of experts in gross anatomy, microscopic anatomy, embryology, osteology, paleoanthropology, and to the graduate students and the anatomy lab crew, two weeks prior to the first day of instruction of the incoming second year class. Paired off in groups of two, the six table docs were given three cadavers to dissect plus copies of *Man's Anatomy*, Tobias's practical dissection manual. Filled with a rich array of systems, scored with a practical description of how to dissect from the skin inwards, in a rational, disciplined way, like a map showing where to go next, the three volumes were divided into extremities, thorax and abdomen, and head and neck, with cross references and an index that was easy to follow. Almost every page was enriched by simple line diagrams of muscles, organs, bones, arteries, veins, and nerves. The diagrams of muscles showed their attachments to bones, and accompanying descriptions detailed their relationships to other muscles, organs, bones, joints, and nerves and identified what movements were produced by contracting the muscle. I had used the exact same dissection manual as a medical student.

I oversaw twenty-eight medical students, and since I was only slightly ahead of them in dissecting the same part of the body, following Tobias's manual, I appeared to be a source of remarkable knowledge while I repeated every step seven times with each group of four students per cadaver. Enjoying my depth of knowledge, focusing on remembering vast numbers of facts, I quickly became the source of help for my students, filled with youthful inquisitiveness and a never-ending array of questions.

The medical school was filled with brilliant academics, and Tobias himself, a brilliant "Renaissance man," teacher, scientist, and administrator, demanded unrelenting attention to perfection. My creative and curious side, continually aimed at discovering something new, drew me into a research project with Tobias that involved examining the teeth of ancient fossils, comparing molar tooth development from the hominid ancestors of Man that had been excavated from anthropological sites in Southern Africa. He instructed John, a Canadian post-doctoral fellow from Hamilton, Ontario. I volunteered to help, much to the surprise of my fellow table docs who were embedded, as was I, in learning so much detailed anatomy while also studying physiology and pathology, all very time consuming. My brain rebelled at the robot-like intake of facts, and I needed the opportunity to exercise my research brain. My colleagues thought I would stray from my main goal of passing the primary exam, but I knew from my research experience in medical school that I had enough discipline and tenacity to accomplish both.

Tobias approached every project, every new problem, with the energy, intention, knowledge, and anticipation of an army general planning a major military exercise. The experiment involved microscopic measuring of tooth cusp surfaces. The technicians measuring the bumps and ridges, including me, were required to make detailed observations. The project was important in the understanding of the origins of Man.

Obsessive in everything he did, not satisfied to just send us into the storage facilities to examine anthropological artifacts, Tobias micromanaged the measurements of every case. He watched as I set up the calipers, magnifying glasses, microscopes, and the lab recording books.

"Remember to take three readings at each of three sites."

I already knew this because he had taken all the "technicians" through the protocol, but it reminded me that accurate observation depends upon careful execution and razor-sharp scrutiny. That attention to detail is what made Tobias a world-renowned scientist. Louis Leakey, the world famous British paleoanthropologist and archaeologist whose work in Olduvai Gorge in East Africa was important in demonstrating that humans evolved in Africa, entrusted Tobias to do the vital and detailed analysis of the first tooth and other fossilized bones of a new tool-using hominid species, *Homo habilis*, or "handyman," thought at the time to be an intermediary between the gracile *Australopithecus*, identified by Tobias's teacher in Johannesburg, Raymond Dart, and modern man. Tobias's complicated book on the rich details of *Homo habilis'* anatomy won international respect, and it was rumored that he was on the short list for a Nobel Prize for his discoveries and reporting of the Origins of Man in Africa.

A little intimidated by Tobias watching every move I made, I moved the calipers deliberately, recording the numbers in a lab book specially designed for the project. More than once he urged me to move the probe a little more anterior, or a little more posterior, or even inferior or superior, until he was absolutely satisfied that I was in the right place and I recorded the findings accurately. It was exhausting, but I was reminded of my photographic dark room experiences as a child and my sickle cell thalassemia study as a medical student. Science requires accurate observation and absolute honesty in analyzing the data obtained. Sloppy observation would result in incorrect conclusions.

A visit to an anthropological digging site, Makapansgat, in the Northern Transvaal province near Potgietersrust with Tobias and a team of paleoanthropologists all intent on the tedious job of brushing and gently chiseling Brescia off two million-year-old animal bones from the caves, gave me additional insight into the process of scientific discovery. Tobias frequently showed his hawk-like ability to see things that others in the party failed to see. Walking toward the mountains from our campsite in the valley one day, he suddenly stopped on the flat grassland path and, using a small spade, leaned forward and dug something out of the ground. It was a fossilized mouse skeleton which no one else had seen. Like a child presented with a long-sought gift, he animatedly described how a swooping hawk would have grabbed a small animal and swallowed it whole. Sometime later, the hawk regurgitated the skeletal remains, the rest digested inside the bird, and the small bones would undergo the fossilization process that ancient hominid and other animal bones had undergone inside the caves.

"How did you see something so small that no one else saw?" I asked.

"Remember one of Louis Pasteur's favorite aphorisms: in the fields of observation, chance favors only the prepared mind."

"That is powerful. I guess that means that a relatively inexperienced young man cannot see important details until he has a lot of knowledge and experience. Do you think it possible for someone like me to make original observations and come up with new knowledge?"

"You need confidence while you explore the world, recognizing that we don't yet know all the secrets of the universe. Just remember that whatever field you find yourself, don't be discouraged by the skepticism of experts. Live in the serene peace of laboratories and libraries. It is in those places that you will grow, strengthen, and improve, and where you will learn to study and understand the works of nature. Whether your efforts are or are not favored by life, you should be able to say, when you come near your great goal, 'I have done what I could.'"

"Does that mean I need a laboratory to create new knowledge?" I asked.

"I believe there is a difference between those who do extensive research in laboratories, using the Enlightenment ideas developed in seventeenth century Western Europe, and those who use deductive reasoning popularized by Aristotle in Ancient Greece. For Aristotelian science, you need to observe, record, and come to logical conclusions. We see examples of that in many walks of life, and it may have some value, although a lot of the logic is based upon unproven truths. Modern laboratory research, and I include our vast laboratory here at Makapansgat, a laboratory without walls, asks that we start with a hypothesis, based on proven facts, with the aim of advancing knowledge further. The experiments we do to prove the hypothesis, when carefully designed and executed, require knowledge, curiosity, careful observation, and thoughtful analysis. You have the makings of a fine researcher, and you'll need to think carefully whether you really want to complete training in general surgery after your year with us."

Startled by this comment, I started to think about what it might mean for my future. It seemed like he was telling me that he had seen some promise in my need to do research, probably when I assisted him with the hominid tooth studies. I wanted to be a surgeon, and that was the main reason for me to take a year out to teach anatomy. I had not come into the anatomy department intending to learn research. But he sensed my inquisitive nature and my unrelenting curiosity. Perhaps I could not only train to become a competent surgeon but also use my knowledge and curiosity to do research in surgery.

Training eyes to see, ears to listen, hands to feel, and noses to smell and connecting those observations to an alert brain, the basis of any scientist's toolbox to make an experiment come alive, would also be helpful to my learning great details of the anatomy of the human body and to discover new information.

One of my medical students asked me a difficult question:

"We learn about all the systems of the body, and we can see them as we dissect the cadaver. But when we look for lymphatic vessels, we can't find them. How do anatomists know where the lymphatics are if they can't see them in a cadaver, and surgeons apparently can't see them during operations?"

I remembered my repeated exposure to the lymphatic system, starting as an eleven-year-old boy in the Johannesburg Public Library, and then again as a fifteen year old when my grandmother had Hodgkin's disease, and again in the morgue during an autopsy on a young woman with Hodgkin's disease, and my experience with Professor DuPlessis when he told me the lymph node in my neck did not need a biopsy, and in my internship year when I assisted surgeons removing lymph nodes from the neck, armpits, groins, abdomen, and chest. Lymph nodes, part of the lymphatic system, are found in defined anatomic sites, but the little "tubes" that lead to and from them, the lymphatic trunks, are colorless, tiny, and invisible.

Found in clusters throughout the human body, lymph nodes are tiny, bean-shaped structures connected to each other by a large network of lymphatic vessels, a connecting series of anatomically sophisticated thin-walled tubes concealed from the naked eye. These tiny lymphatic vessels transport lymph, a clear fluid generated from the circulatory system in the tissues of the body to the nearest lymph nodes, in clusters in the neck, armpit, groin, and a few other places. The lymph fluid passes through multiple lymph nodes and eventually passes back into the blood stream.

"Let's do a little research together and find out how those lymphatics were discovered and how we can be sure that lymph, the clear cell-free fluid that runs in those lymphatics, drains the way that the textbooks say. Come back tomorrow and let me know how far you went with the question."

We discovered that the first lymphatics were discovered by Gaspare Aselli who found vessels filled with a white fluid around the small intestine of a living well-fed dog in 1622, calling them "lacteals," or milky veins. These vessels were invisible in dogs who had been starved before dissection. He wrote about this finding in a booklet in 1627, and the resultant rush to dissection and vivisection of hundreds of animals resulted in what was called "lymphomania."

Sappey, a nineteenth century French anatomist, devised a procedure to define and delineate the lymphatic system by injecting mercury into the skin of a cadaver in order to properly view the individual lymphatic vessels and, in 1874, published an anatomical atlas, drawn by his wife, Antoinette, that included a detailed study of lymph draining from the skin through tiny tubes, or vessels, into lymph nodes in the neck, armpit, and groin and from those nodes back to the bloodstream and to the heart.

The heart pumps about twenty liters of blood around the body through blood vessels every day. The blood vessel capillaries, the smallest of the blood vessels, not only transport seventeen liters of blood directly into the veins and back to the heart, they also filter the blood into the tissues between blood vessels, producing about three liters of interstitial fluid plasma per day that carries nutrients to the cells, collects waste products, bacteria, and damaged cells, and then drains as lymph via a sizeable network of lymphatic vessels back towards the heart, filtered on the way by numerous lymph nodes. The lymphatic system may be like a modern police force, constantly watching people, looking for suggestive information, sometimes using facial recognition, or fingerprints, or DNA analysis, or GPS signals from personal cell phones to find criminals, and mobilizing members of the force to stop potential damage to vulnerable individuals or property by incarceration, the prison system mimicking the ability of the immune system to stop dangerous infections by a sort of cordoning-off process in the tissues.

Fascinated by the extra reading and library research produced by his question to me, the student next asked me about breast cancer.

"My aunt had a radical mastectomy for breast cancer, and she developed a swollen arm. I noticed this when I was just a kid, and you couldn't miss it. Her arm was so big she couldn't get it through the sleeves of her dress or jackets. She had to enlarge her clothes to be able to wear them. Have you ever seen this?"

"Sure. That's called lymphedema. Radical mastectomy is sometimes done for breast cancer. It is an operation where the breast, all the axillary lymph nodes, and the pectoral muscles between those two structures are removed. The swelling occurs in the arm because the lymph that normally drains through the axillary lymph nodes is blocked and dams back into the arm. It is a difficult problem and is chronic, and incurable."

"I can understand why the breast and the axillary nodes are removed. But why are the pectoral muscles removed?"

"Because the lymphatics that drain the breast go through the muscle."

"I don't think Sappey showed that in his atlas. Besides, lymphatics don't seem to go through muscles anywhere else in the body. Or do they? I'm not certain."

"You have a point. Let's give ourselves another project in the library. Let's see if there is definitive evidence that lymphatics traverse the pectoral muscles."

"Okay."

The key issue was the question of whether lymphatics from the breast pass through the pectoral muscles to get to the axillary lymph nodes lodged behind the muscle. Two papers by Gray in the late 1930s provided the proof that my student and I needed. Using injection techniques like those used by Sappey in the nineteenth century, Gray showed that lymphatics draining fluid from the breast did not go through the pectoral muscle. Instead, they followed a superficial route around the muscle into the axilla.

The devastation of radical mastectomy, visible in women with swollen arms, clearly evident ribs, and an absent breast, was obvious to me when I had seen patients who had that operation, but my surgical teachers seemed quite unfeeling with women who suffered from the lifelong complications and side effects of the procedure. Surgeons justified the operation by saying it cured many patients and that patients should be grateful that they were alive, even though they had altered anatomic and psychological status because of the operation. Now it seemed to me that the original premise of the operation, first popularized in the late nineteenth century by William Halsted in Baltimore, was based on the belief that lymphatics passed through the pectoral muscles, a belief proven false fifty years later.

Upon further library research, I found that others had come to the same conclusion as I had. In a 1948 paper, Patey and Dyson in England reported their thirteen-year experience with a modified mastectomy that preserved the pectoral muscles compared to the standard radical mastectomy. They found no difference in survival or local recurrence rates between the two groups.

"This information is very important," I said.

"How come it took so many years for so many people involved in treating breast cancer to recognize that an operation, based on an anatomically false belief, was way too radical and resulted in so many women suffering irreparable harm?"

"Your question is obviously important. But if you look back at the history of gross anatomy, the kind that we know these days, the kind of anatomy that you're learning now, where you can take Tobias's book and dissect and find exactly what is in the book, repeated in every cadaver in the anatomy lab, we sort of take that truth for granted. But think about the anatomy that earlier physicians knew, based on illustrations in books, in drawings going back almost two thousand years from the Greek physician Galen in the second century AD, based on animal vivisection, perpetuated and unchallenged for thirteen hundred years by generation upon generation of physicians until Vesalius in the 16th century. Vesalius, during public dissections in Padua of executed criminals, showed that the anatomy of humans was different from that of monkeys. His superbly executed drawings in his treatise *De humani corporis fabrica*, challenged Galen "drawing for drawing." His are triumphant descriptions of the differences between animals and humans, but it took a further century for Galen's influence to fade. Vesalius's work marked a new era in the study of anatomy and its relation to medicine. Under Vesalius, anatomy became an actual discipline."

"Is that why we honor him by naming our anatomy lecture hall as 'the Vesalian?'"

"Yes, I believe so. The lesson from your questions is that we should always be open to being surprised. It is good to challenge, question, and explore every opinion you come across—especially your own."

Ideas might begin innocently enough, but like garden weeds, they can sometimes grow relentlessly and overtake everything else. I kept thinking about the origin and development of scientific facts and slowly realized that my repeated exposure to lymphatics, lymph nodes, the immune system, and the way one generation might believe in a "fact" as being the incontrovertible truth would often result in new knowledge in a later generation that overturned that "fact."

CHAPTER 8

DARWIN AND THE UNSEEN

Scientific endeavors in the anatomy department, influenced by Tobias and his predecessor Raymond Dart, heavily dependent upon ideas, knowledge, and scientific truth, fed my soul more than anything I had learned in medical school. Every day, while learning and teaching facts, and based on how supposedly true facts had affected the development of a terrible operation for breast cancer, based upon a false understanding of human anatomy and physiology, I realized that I was turned on to challenge truths in my future surgical life.

Breathing the same air as the graduate students and academic staff, influenced by the daily excitement of new questions, eating lunch in the staff recreation room, and talking about new ideas made me realize more and more that my mind was turned on by the ways of looking at the origins of Man, and very soon, I started to wonder about how Darwin had come up with the ideas of evolution and natural selection.

I vaguely knew about Darwin and his revolutionary book *The Origin of Species*, published in 1859, but at that time, Darwinism was not taught in high schools or to medical students. When Tobias offered a series of eight lectures on Charles Darwin to his graduate students, I jumped at the opportunity to attend, even though the time spent and the reading necessary diluted my time learning and teaching anatomy.

The ideas of natural selection were critically important in the department because of the very nature of paleoanthropology, a branch of paleontology with a human focus which seeks to understand the early development of anatomically modern humans through the reconstruction of evolutionary kinship lines within the family Hominidae, working from biological evidence (such as petrified skeletal remains, bone fragments, footprints) and cultural evidence (such as stone tools, artifacts, and settlement localities).

Tobias's lectures were like listening to a Shakespearean actor on a stage, his voice clear, vigorous, and melodious, his gestures vivid, his ideas and thought sequences stunningly logical, making the difficult easy, his thoughts peppered with stories of people making the science more human. Putting Darwin's ideas into a realistic relationship with his own department, he told many stories about Professor Dart, the first chairman of our anatomy department and Tobias's teacher, friend, and colleague for many years, who had become world famous because of his discovery and naming of a new species of hominin, *Australopithecus Africanus*, a bipedal human ancestor, a transitional form between ape and human.

In keeping with his flair for the dramatic, and his love of stories, Tobias began the series of lectures by telling the story of the Piltdown Man, based on a fossil discovered at a construction site in England in 1912 and thought initially to represent an evolutionary missing link between apes and humans but eventually proven to be a hoax perpetrated by an amateur archeologist. When Dart published his findings in 1924 of the first Australopithecine fossil found at Taung, the world of paleoanthropology was still reeling from the Piltdown deception, and the discovery was discarded by European scientists. It took twenty years for prominent English paleoanthropologists to acknowledge that they had been wrong, and Dart correct in his assessment of the "missing link," a term stimulated by Darwin's observations.

Darwin's discoveries were described in detail, flavored with rich personal stories. Tobias favored examples that exemplified how Darwin worked, why his methods were worth emulating, how he found unique science even in as simple a place as his own garden, which led to a book on garden worms.

He emphasized the value of caution in publishing but admonished us all to be aware that other scientists might beat us to publication if we remained too cautious.

Darwin was almost eclipsed by Alfred Russel Wallace who had worked for years in the Amazon Basin, Indonesia, and Australasia and who independently conceived the theory of evolution through natural selection. This information prompted Darwin to publish his own ideas in *On the Origin of Species* when he realized that Wallace had come to conclusions similar to his own, ideas that started twenty-eight years previously during his voyage on the Beagle.

"Darwin's scientific discovery is the unifying theory of the life sciences, explaining the diversity of life," said Tobias. "I know you're aware of his work and findings while exploring the Galapagos Islands in the Pacific Ocean off the coast of South America. That area has become popular for people to visit. His observations on differing beak morphology of mockingbirds and finches, differing slightly from island to island, and differing from similar birds in Chile, certainly helped him conceive his theory of natural selection. But I want to make sure you recognize the immensity of his imagination and the continuing interest in doing research, asking questions, and writing about his mental meanderings. He examined human origins, evolution, transmutation of species, sexual selection, plants, the formation of vegetable mold through the action of worms, the descent of Man, the marsupial rat-kangaroo, the platypus, and Aborigines in Australia, tortoises, the geology of South America, sea shells on mountain tops, emotions in Man and animals, and many other topics. He had a voracious and insatiable appetite for questioning and observing anything and everything. That is the story of a scientist."

I was most interested in Tobias's interpretations of the support given to Darwin by his friend Thomas Huxley, particularly in dealing with the religious dogmas by church leaders in England at the time, and by antagonistic rivals like Wilberforce, whose sarcastic retorts about Man arising from apes led to public rhetoric and endless cartoons in daily newspapers in London. There was certainly no uniform acceptance of the concept of natural selection, although most people accepted that there was some form of evolution in biology.

I had my own issues with religion and dogmas, having come across many people in my family and in my neighborhood whose ideas were often generated by scientifically unproven beliefs and based on faith. Huxley and Darwin promoted science, pure and free, untrammeled by religious dogmas. They campaigned pugnaciously against the authority of the clergy in education, aiming to overturn the dominance of clergymen and aristocratic amateurs in favor of a new generation of professional scientists.

My thoughts turned to the nature of scientific discovery. Tobias's lecture series gave me an idea about the concealed truths in the world around me. Evolution and natural selection are clearly apparent to us these days, but those artifacts and observations that led Darwin to his conclusions had been there for eons but unrecognized by millions of people until he drew attention to them. Now the ideas are revealed whereas before they were concealed and unknown. This is true of most discoveries, as clearly evidenced by many daily events that we now take for granted, such as automobiles, airplanes, microbes, insulin for diabetes, antibiotics for bacterial infections, prevention of surgical site infections by antisepsis, computers, blood transfusions, insecticides, and rockets to the moon, all of these inventions changing the way we live, adding to the ease of living and to our happiness, and which we can easily see.

The pursuit of truth remains at the heart of scientific endeavor. Truth matters in science. Truth in science is not esoteric dilly-dallying. It shapes climate science, medicine, public health, the economy, and many other worldly endeavors. Tobias asked us to think about ideas in science which were found to be wrong because of careful questioning of the validity of beliefs, some of which had become part of the daily understanding of life by the vast majority of people.

He asked us to consider Ptolemy's geocentric model of the universe, the predominant description of the cosmos in many ancient civilizations, based on the belief that the sun, moon, and planets orbited the earth, an idea supported by scientists at that time observing the sun, the moon, stars, and the planets revolving around the earth once a day. To earthbound observers, the earth felt solid, stable, and stationary. Those ideas seemed obvious, and they held sway for over 1,500 years until gradually superseded, with much resistance by Christian theologians to the transition, by the heliocentric model of Copernicus, Galileo, and Kepler of planets revolving around the sun, which we now know to be "true."

Tobias then drew our attention to phlogiston, a fictional imponderable fluid that natural philosophers at the time believed was a necessary ingredient during combustion, which disappeared from the lexicon when Lavoisier, using scientific experiments, discovered oxygen, the true ingredient necessary for fire.

"Think about how Darwin has affected your life when you sit down to think through new experiments. I hope his life and works will provide fuel for you at just the right moment. I hope you already have hearts and minds consumed by the fire of seeking new knowledge."

Teaching provided the stimulus for me to be so adept in anatomy that there was no part of the body that I didn't know "inside out." Passing the Primary examination of the College of Surgeons was a breeze.

The atmosphere in the anatomy department under the watchful eyes of Philip Tobias was a big extra stimulus for my restless need to discover. I was already consumed by the need to "see the unseen" in the world, having experienced the joy of developing pictures in the photographic darkroom and my exciting diagnostic and research efforts in sickle cell thalassemia. My year of teaching anatomy and doing research with Tobias came to an end with me ready to enter the next phase of my life, learning surgery, pursuing the unseen lymphatics and any other area that was concealed.

Chapter 9

Seeing

Returning to Coronation Hospital as a mid-level surgical trainee five years after my meaningful diagnosis of sickle cell thalassemia as a medical student, and a year after passing the primary examination of the college of surgeons, a year filled with piling facts into my brain and techniques into my hands and learning how to connect the two, and still believing that I was destined to discover something unique, I was hungry to uncover new ideas but bound by an understanding that I could not innovate without mastering the basic knowledge in the discipline.

Each new encounter with patients had the potential to introduce me to a disease I may never previously have seen. Most of the cases were common and straight forward, what we called "textbook cases." But some were more challenging, such as the massive esophageal bypass surgeries for esophageal stricture caused by drinking lye. For some psychological, sociological, or cultural reason, swallowing the highly caustic fluid used for cleaning kitchens and homes was the method of choice for attempting suicide by women in Coronationville. Some died from this poison, but those who didn't die were destined to end up with caustic strictures of the esophagus, and we saw them as emaciated, unhappy, usually young women with rubber tubes inserted into their stomachs for feeding because they couldn't swallow food. They came to Tanne, one of the two surgical chiefs, because he had undertaken to help many of these women by doing an operation that took eight hours to complete and consisted of connecting the stomach to the neck with a long piece of the large intestine placed through the chest and connected to the esophagus in the neck. When this difficult operation worked well, the resulting emotional rebound of the patients was astounding, because they could once more swallow food.

Reading the topic of caustic strictures of the esophagus in the textbook, I found there were other methods to manage the disease. I asked Tanne whether he had published anything on the operation he did for these patients. He had not.

"Wouldn't it be valuable to report your experience?" I asked.

He smiled and said: "This is a well described operation. I'm just doing the procedure that others have described."

"Have you thought about developing a new approach to the management of this disease?"

"I believe one should not try to change something that is working well."

Still early in my training, I realized that I should learn and master the standard approaches to all the common operations. But, after this conversation, I was disappointed with the possibility that I, too, might one day lose the thrill of innovation, of developing new and better approaches to surgical diseases.

Boris Lewin and David Tanne, the two attending general surgical chiefs, were available during the daytime to discuss cases. At night, when they were not around, I had my surgery textbook to consult. Neither Tanne nor Lewin came to the hospital at night, expecting me and two interns to take care of some complex issues which I was nowhere near competent in managing. I knew that I could call them if I had a question.

Confronted with a young man who had stepped in front of a speeding car one night, I used my textbook and my memory to initiate the resuscitation and management of the trauma. The only major injury this patient had was a stable fractured pelvis. I went through all the motions of management, the so-called "ABCs," and discovered I could not pass a Foley catheter through his penis into the bladder. When I tried, I discovered a drop of blood at the tip of the penis. Having just completed a four-month rotation in urology, I quickly realized this patient had a ruptured urethra, caused by the shearing force of the pubic bone at the level of the prostate gland by the impact of the car. I had never seen a case like this but vaguely knew how this injury could be repaired, and since we had no urologist on call, I called Tanne.

"Take the patient to the operating room, prepare him for a lower abdominal incision, and call me when you're ready."

Two hours later, with the patient prepared with sterile solution, and draped in a sterile way, I had the nurse call Tanne and put the telephone up to my ear.

"I'm ready for you, sir," I said.

"Okay. Make a midline incision, open the abdomen, do a careful inspection and make sure he doesn't have any ruptured organs other than the urethra, and then call me back."

Stunned, because I realized I was on my own, taking responsibility for an operation with minimal prior experience, I did as I was bid.

The nurse called Tanne again.

"What did you find? Is the bladder intact?"

"Yes, sir. But it seems to be floating free, away from the pubis."

"Good. You made the correct diagnosis. Now, the next part is a little tricky, so listen carefully. Make an incision in the bladder and find the opening for the urethra and pass a ten French catheter through into the space where the prostate gland has sheared off at the pubis. You will see the tip of the catheter. Then pass a sixteen French Foley catheter with a ten-milliliter bulb through the penis into that same space and sew the tips of the two catheters together with heavy silk suture. Then gently pull the bladder catheter back into the bladder while at the same time pushing the penile catheter towards the bladder. Once that Foley is in the bladder, remove the silk suture and the first catheter, inflate the bulb of the Foley with ten milliliters of sterile saline, and pull back until the ruptured ends of the urethra are approximated. Call me back when you're done."

About thirty minutes later, the nurse called Tanne again.

"How did that work out for you?" he asked.

"It seems to have worked, sir."

"Good. Now you need to place a few catgut sutures in the ends of the urethra to help keep those ends approximated. Start by pulling the bladder and prostate away from the pubis, place about four sutures through the wall of the urethra on both sides; keep the sutures long, don't tie them down, but keep them clamped and ready until all the sutures have been placed. Then pull the prostate back down using the Foley catheter and then tie down the sutures. Call me when that is done."

That part took another thirty minutes, and the nurse called Tanne again.

"Are you done?" he asked.

"Yes, sir."

"Good. Now just close the bladder in two layers, put a couple of sutures through the bladder wall, and snug them to the periosteum of the pubis, close the abdomen like we usually do and take the patient back to the ward when he's awake. The important part of this repair is that you need to keep a two-pound weight on a pulley, keeping tension on the Foley catheter for at least five days. I'll see you in the morning."

Over the next few days, while watching the patient carefully, I researched articles and books in the library and discovered there were many other ways of treating this kind of injury in the operating room. They all seemed to work according to the surgeons who described them. No one had done scientific studies to compare them to each other. I had a new feeling, when the patient was able to pee normally, and we took the Foley catheter out. I felt a surging pride, a triumph that reminded me how I had felt when I made my first photographic enlargement and when I diagnosed sickle cell thalassemia on the patient that led to my winning the research prize as a medical student. That feeling was so wonderful, so addictive, that I wanted it all the time.

I felt exhilarated every time an operation resulted in a cure. A young adult male came in with severe pain in the abdomen, made worse by walking or even climbing up on the examining table in the emergency room. We operated and took out the ruptured appendix, and he improved dramatically. The change in his pain and his mood, the way he looked at me when he thanked me, put me in an extremely good mood. I smiled a lot, felt like everyone admired me, and I felt like a hero. Appendicitis before the introduction of antibiotics was not always curable. Even in the early twentieth century, before the advances in anesthesia and modern-day operating room gadgets, young, healthy people died of the disease. In 1834 Sir John Ericksen, surgeon to Queen Victoria, strongly believed that smart and wise surgeons would not operate on the abdomen because it was too dangerous; how many people with appendicitis without surgery in those days survived? Now we operated on the abdomen, chest, and brain every day in our modern hospitals, thousands of patients every year with relatively few complications.

Fascinated by the advances in medicine, I set myself a task of discovering the contributions of surgical innovators. Surgical innovation, different from basic science research which does not necessarily require application or have an intended use, introduces something new, usually a new idea or a new method, something thought up or mentally imagined, has a rich tradition and one which has been fundamental to surgical progress. As one of the oldest and most respected fields, surgery has had a unique culture and deep tradition built upon continuous innovation. Most of the innovations in surgery were because of creating new or modifying existing tools or creating new technologies, such as hemodialysis, organ transplantation, cardio-pulmonary bypass, artificial heart valves, artificial blood vessels, pacemakers, mechanical joint replacements, anesthesia, antisepsis, blood transfusion, laparoscopy, and robotic surgery.

I had come to realize that most surgeons innovate daily, adapting therapies and operations to the basic distinctiveness of every patient and their disease, stimulated by repetitive failures of existing therapies or by unsolved problems. In fact, surgeons face clinical decisions on an hourly basis, many with substantial influence and outcome. My own training required daily situation assessment, decision analysis, and a frequent development of new processes. Each clinical case offered unique challenges and required a degree of creativity.

The eighteenth-century surgical innovator, John Hunter, was an early advocate of careful observation and scientific method in medicine. A teacher and collaborator of Edward Jenner, pioneer of the smallpox vaccine, he became an authority of many subjects, including human teeth, bone growth and remodeling, inflammation, gunshot wounds, venereal diseases, digestion, the functioning of the lacteals, child development, the separateness of maternal and fetal blood supplies, and the role of the lymphatic system. The lymphatic system studies caught my attention, and I found that Hunter was an inveterate collector of human and animal specimens and had perhaps even injected himself with tissues from an executed felon who suffered syphilis and gonorrhea.

I imagined what he must have felt when he made new discoveries, like the first tooth transplant, and the excitement of discovery was always present in me when I read stories of Hunter and other surgical innovators.

One of my most dazzling experiences as a final year medical student had occurred in August 1966. Bert Myburgh, an energetic Rhodes scholar, a brilliant, inspiring, good-looking, athletic, academic surgeon, with the help of American transplant pioneer Thomas Starzl, did the first kidney transplant in South Africa at the Johannesburg General Hospital. The kidney was removed from one person and put into another, and after the vein, artery, and ureter were connected, it was magical to see the new kidney become pink and produce urine in the recipient. Like a mesmerized puppy dog, I followed Myburgh around, watching him do organ transplants in baboons on the seventh floor of the medical school, and in patients in the hospital, always listening carefully to the hypnotic cadence of his professorial teaching on ward rounds and in the lecture hall, and deciding right there that I wanted to be just like him.

Those years were filled with innovation. South Africa, and the rest of the world, was awakened to a new era in medicine in December 1967, just as I was completing my first post-graduate training year, by a human heart transplant in Louis Washkansky, a fifty-four-year-old grocer who was suffering from diabetes and incurable heart disease in Cape Town, a thousand miles southwest of Johannesburg, by Christiaan Barnard, chief of cardio-thoracic surgery at Groote Schuur Hospital. I had met the famous heart surgeon during my trip to the Association of Medical Students of South Africa conference in 1965, when he gave me the award for best medical student research paper on stage in a large auditorium.

During a training rotation at the Transvaal Memorial Hospital for children in 1969, when I operated on a newborn infant with intestinal atresia, I discovered that Barnard, as a young doctor experimenting on dogs, was able to reproduce this condition in a fetus puppy by tying off some of the blood supply to the puppy's intestines and then placing the animal back in the womb, after which it was born some two weeks later with the condition of intestinal atresia. He had developed a remedy for this defect that had saved the lives of many babies around the world. He had studied and published on tuberculous meningitis, always lethal until the advent of streptomycin treatment in the

1940s. The more I read about him, the more I realized the pattern of his restless curiosity and creativity, a trend that I recognized in other innovators, and in myself.

What is innovation, and how is it best encouraged? Far from sudden "eureka" moments, innovation is almost always a gradual process, advancing by small incremental steps, often conducted by teams of people. Any innovative idea is likely to come from several individuals, such as the invention of the lightbulb, the idea for which was proposed by dozens of people independently before Thomas Edison produced one which worked and revolutionized lighting around the world. Charles Townes, winner of the Nobel Prize in physics for his discovery of lasers, liked telling the story of a rabbit and a beaver looking up at the Hoover Dam. The beaver said he didn't invent the dam, but it came from his idea. The Gates Foundation has encouraged innovation in Africa that saved hundreds of thousands of lives from malaria and pneumococcal pneumonia.

I was on the lookout for innovative ideas.

Operating at Coronation Hospital with Boris Lewin, a loud-mouthed, chain-smoking, large bear of a man with enormous hands and a foreign accent, was almost always entertaining because of his gruff technique and questions demanding that I stay alert. Removal of part of the thyroid gland in the neck, most often done for tumors or over production of thyroid hormone, a delicate procedure requiring a detailed knowledge of the anatomy of nerves, arteries, the parathyroid glands, and the larynx, seemed rather incongruous with the indelicate Boris wielding the scalpels, scissors, forceps, clamps, and needle holders. Not expecting to be stimulated to think deeply or creatively with him, expecting to do surgical procedures with manly efficiency, I was surprised one day, in the middle of a thyroid operation, to see that I had underestimated his surgical intellect. There appeared to be a separate nodule of pink solid tissue on one side of the thyroid gland, which I thought was a lymph node.

"What is that nodule lateral to the main thyroid gland?" asked Lewin.

"It looks to me like a metastasis to a lymph node," I answered.

"Ha! That's what most people used to say. This is a lateral aberrant thyroid. Look at this flimsy connection between the two."

He was right, and I remained amazed as he delicately removed both the main gland and the lateral piece plus the intervening tissue in one piece.

"Take a picture of that specimen," he instructed. "This is a very rare condition, and I want you to do a little reading and present the case to the entire surgery staff at the Johannesburg General Hospital at Grand Rounds next week. Pay particular attention to the embryologic development of the thyroid."

Given an instruction like that turned on my library research brain, and I found articles that helped explain the aberrant embryologic origins of the thyroid gland in the embryo. Having done library research and written reports and papers on various topics, I quickly had a slick slide presentation ready to be delivered to the entire Johannesburg surgical community. I was very nervous.

"Don't worry so much," Lewin said. "When you stand at that lectern on Saturday, just remember you know more about this rare topic than anyone else in the room."

The experience of doing my first presentation in that imposing auditorium in front of the chairman of the Surgery Department, Professor D J DuPlessis, called "Sonny" by his friends, "Dup" by many of us, or "God" by many who had suffered his immense presence, and scathing personal, derogatory comments, required me to bring together all my years of performing in front of audiences, in classrooms at school, in teaching anatomy in Tobias's department, on the sports fields while playing important competitive matches, and presenting cases to the team on ward rounds. I didn't realize that Lewin had deliberately planned for me to give this presentation because it was like a job interview.

The aim of every surgical trainee at Coronation Hospital, and Baragwanath, the other "non-white" hospital in apartheid South Africa, was to be called to train in DuPlessis's prestigious surgical circuit at the Johannesburg General Hospital, an academic opportunity second to none in Africa and, as I came to realize after moving to the United States, amongst the best in the world. I received the call from the professor one day, and he offered me the position, spent thirty minutes telling me that it would be easier to replace me than to replace a nurse, advising me that my job was to learn, to take care of his patients, become a safe surgeon, and be alert to bringing new knowledge to the world.

My opportunity began in 1970.

Chapter 10

Advanced Learning

DuPlessis not only ran the surgery department of Wits medical school, but he seemed to also control the entire Johannesburg General Hospital, also known as the "gen." Having been appointed to his position at age forty in 1958, after serving in the South African army in North Africa during World War II, one of the youngest heads of department in the history of the school, he had already trained thirty-six general surgeons by the time I started in his training circuit in 1970. He was so powerful that even the chairman of the internal medicine department seemed to accede to his demands.

Every surgical unit at the "gen" was managed like a military outfit, starting from the uniforms. We all wore spotless white coats, short haircuts, white shirts with ties, long flannel pants, and highly polished leather shoes. There were no women doctors training or on the faculty. We were never late for rounds on patients, the operating rooms, or lectures. The hierarchy of surgical trainees and teachers was rigidly enforced, and I could not go directly to the chief with any issue unless I had an acute emergency with one of his patients. Weekly working hours were always somewhere in the region of one hundred. Sleep was something babies and old people did, not us. Personally derogatory reprimand, like the kinds used by sergeant majors in the army, was a daily occurrence. Questions were allowed but only if they were sensible, intelligent, and stated in the most truncated form. Naïve or "stupid" questions were ridiculed.

Military style, no excuses were allowed.

My goal as I entered the "Dup" circuit was to shine as a clinician and to find an area of research that would allow me to shine as an academic surgeon. "Dup" himself was a world-renowned expert in peptic ulcers of the stomach and duodenum. He had unlimited access to the marvelously equipped animal facilities on the seventh floor of the medical school where Buddy Lawson, one of his mentees, did most of the ulcer research on dogs and pigs. We did a lot of stomach ulcer surgeries on patients and, when we removed most or all the stomach, part of the experimental protocol was to roll the tissues like a Swiss roll so that the research pathologist could make histology slides and look at vast swaths of the lining of the stomach all at once. "Dup" believed that back flow of bile from the duodenum into the stomach caused chronic inflammation of the stomach lining and that was the precursor of stomach ulcers. Mapping the area of chronic inflammation and the areas where ulcers were found was one piece of evidence for his hypothesis.

The ulcer research excited me, and I could identify with the extensive layout and investigative capabilities of the surgery department. My prior efforts to seek answers in my home photographic lab, and in Stein's Clinical Pathology lab, and my ongoing library research talent gave me the necessary skills and perceptive abilities to recognize possible defects in the vast database that filled five-foot high metal filing cabinets in Dup's office that contained slides and clinical information on every case.

Looking at research on stomach ulcers in the rest of the world gave me my first insights into how "Dup's" research might have been wrong. I discovered that Buddy Lawson had connected the gallbladder to the stomach in dogs and pigs, creating a fistula that leaked bile onto the stomach lining and proved that there was some chronic inflammation in the inner lining around that connection, but he never found ulcers. I thought this was proof enough that the hypothesis could not be correct but, being low on the totem pole, having to prove each day that I was good enough to continue training in general surgery, I had to be careful not to question the chief's ideas. Most experts believed that ulcers in the stomach were associated with chronic inflammation, but no one knew what caused the inflammation until much later when two Australian doctors identified a causative bacterium, H. pylori, for which they won a Nobel Prize.

In "Dup's" ward, I felt like I was in the presence of the "Godfather," as in "Mafia boss" in the movie when I had a question. Somehow it didn't seem like serious and deep questioning of the current dogma on any disease was welcomed, an atmosphere which did not fit well with my forever teeming brain, anxious to question current dogma.

Keeping up with the required reading, with the goal of passing the surgery board exams at the end of my training, I read copiously and carefully enhanced my reading by studying a lot of research papers published in the *British Journal of Surgery*, the *Annals of Surgery*, and a host of other surgery journals from many countries. Becoming more familiar with basic science, remembering my research with Tobias, I noticed that the ideas in "surgical research" seemed to differ from the way scientists set out to answer questions in fields such as paleoanthropology, cell biology, genetics, physics, and biochemistry, so much so that I began to believe that the word "research" associated with "surgery" might have been an incongruity of terms.

Sir Peter Medawar, Nobel laureate, had given a series of six lectures on the philosophy of science at Yale University, and I had just read his published booklet. I came across a page that spoke to the myths of invincibility, superiority, and supposed genius found in powerful departments where groupthink played a powerful role in the ongoing hypothesis, like "Dup's" belief that bile caused gastric ulcers. A graduate student asked Medawar how he could win a Nobel prize. Medawar advised him to find a favorite textbook in his chosen discipline, open any page, read every word very carefully, find the most dogmatic statement, and devote his life to researching that dogma. His advice meant to me that common sense and an inquiring mind are essential to the makeup of a scientist, something which I had already discovered in my early youth.

Regardless of my curious mind, I had to deal with surgical militarism and "manliness." One of my first nights on call had included an emergency operation at 3 a.m., completed at 6 a.m. Hungry, I wolfed down a piece of bread before joining the team at 6:30 for rounds, and meeting "Dup" for the weekly Wednesday teaching rounds in wards twenty-four and twenty-five.

He glared at me and, in front of everybody, asked me why I had not shaved that morning.

"I was operating all night, and I didn't have time to shave," I said.

"That is no excuse," he said, his blue eyes cold and unyielding. Turning to the head nurse he said: "Get him a razor."

Glaring at me, he said: "Don't come back until you're cleaned up."

I sheepishly left, and everyone there knew that they shouldn't gloat or act in any self-righteous way, since it would be their turn sometime to be humiliated.

The training demanded that we look at a world where everything, including every surgery case, could be either black or white or "yes" or "no," not "maybe." There were no grey areas. If a patient came in at 5 a.m. with a set of symptoms and physical signs, it was my job to give "Dup" the definitive diagnosis by 8 a.m. He was so convinced that one only needed two hours or less to come up with the right diagnosis that he would not allow that it was possible to be on the wrong track.

Occasionally, I would have to tell him that I didn't know the diagnosis and therefore could not tell him the plan of treatment. Such was the case when a forty-five-year-old woman came in with sudden abdominal discomfort and in severe shock that required an urgent blood transfusion. The problem was I could not find where she was bleeding. Being quite familiar with patients presenting with shock from bleeding in the gastro-intestinal tract, I had looked for evidence by passing a nasogastric tube into her stomach and testing her stool for blood, but both tests were negative. She had no wounds anywhere, which might have given me a clue since I was quite familiar with severe acute blood loss from penetrating knife wounds or bruising associated with blunt trauma that might point to a ruptured internal organ, like the spleen or the liver. Years later, I could have done a CT scan of the abdomen or placed a needle in the abdomen and aspirated blood after irrigating the peritoneal cavity with saline, but that was not available at that time. I knew she was bleeding from somewhere inside her abdomen but couldn't tell from where. It had to be spontaneous rupture of something. "Dup" asked me what I planned to do with her.

"She needs an operation, sir, and I've booked the operating room."

"What do you plan to do when you've opened her abdomen?" he asked.

"Clean out all the blood and look for the bleeding point."

"Where is that likely to be?"

"It could be anywhere. I will look in all four quadrants and take care of anything that we find."

"Did you look at her abdominal X-ray?" he asked.

"Yes, sir."

"Did you see anything at all that might tell you the diagnosis before you operate?"

"No, sir, I reviewed the X-ray with the radiologist, and there was nothing."

"Let's look at that X-ray together in the doctors' room."

The X-ray film was placed on the X-ray viewing box by the intern. "Dup" sat down in front of this and, pointing with his index finger, he asked: "What do you think of this?"

I couldn't see what he was pointing at.

"Open your eyes; do you see this calcification in the left upper quadrant?"

"Yes, I think I see it now. What is that?"

"If you learn one thing today, it is to keep your eyes open when you look for something. It's no use looking if you don't look carefully. This patient has a ruptured splenic artery aneurysm."

And, without another word, he rose from the chair and walked out the room.

And he was proven right.

As he was most of the time.

Except that he could not see that his bile reflux theory was already disproven by his own staff. The staff could not see that their research disproved the theory. It amazed me to think that one could spend one's entire life in academic surgery, write multiple papers, and not see that one's hypothesis was wrong. Furthermore, he had an entire department of intelligent surgeons who believed his theory and treated patients with gastric ulcers with operations based on a false presumption. Even worse, he gave lectures in other parts of South Africa and in the academic centers of the world to many surgeons, and they might have treated their own patients based upon an incorrect premise.

One day, after returning from the annual conference of the South African Association of Surgeons, Dup sent out an alert to all the surgical trainees in the five academic hospitals under his control demanding that we appear in the departmental lecture room the following day armed with a new research project and a senior mentor. Many of my colleagues in training were not interested in research, but that didn't matter. The resident research prize at the meeting had been won by a resident from a rival medical school, and "Dup" would make sure his trainees would win that prize at every meeting in the future. I called Bert Myburgh and asked if I could work with him on a project. He agreed and introduced me to David Klatzow, a PhD student, who had found a unique protein in the blood of patients dying of cancer.

Working with Klatzow for a few months, during which time we obtained blood samples from dozens of patients with cancer at various stages, and from normal people, and from patients with a host of chronic diseases, we found a consistent pattern of the protein by doing polyacrylamide gel electrophoresis.

That was a time when the world of immunology took a completely new turn, and I thought the protein could be immunosuppressive. The world of immunology was ripe for both basic science and innovation, a time when techniques in transplantation and methods to prevent transplant rejection were studied intensely, a time when I moved to Bert Myburgh's transplantation service to work directly with him.

CHAPTER 11

THE IMMUNE SYSTEM

Learning transplant surgery in the 1970s exposed me to a new era in immunology, an exciting time for surgeons, immunologists, internists, and scientists in general. An understanding of the immune system had developed slowly during the twentieth century, but it was still quite mysterious. The immunology I had learned in medical school focused on serology, cutaneous allergic reactions in children, vaccinations against infectious diseases, and autoimmune diseases. We learned about antibodies that developed against foreign proteins, and the recent elucidation of their structure, just two years before I started medical school. Interferons, a vital group of signaling proteins made and released by host cells in response to the presence of several viruses, were discovered only four years before I started medical school. The cells that most immunologists were interested in were the plasma cells because they made antibodies, uncovered in 1948.

The breakthroughs of various aspects of the immune system were all important, adding small steps without making a universal wall of knowledge until the unearthing of how lymphocytes circulate around the body in 1959. These important cells were found in lymph nodes, the blood, the wall of the intestine, the lungs, spleen, liver, thymus gland, and scattered in other organs, and it was thought that these were the cells that constituted the malignant cells found in Hodgkin's disease, which had peaked my interest when I was a teenager and again as a medical student. However, despite their obvious importance, the role of lymphocytes in the immune responses were not highlighted in our curriculum, and immunology textbooks had sparse information about them.

Bert Myburgh, head of the Transplant Unit within the Department of Surgery, seventeen years older than me, was a bundle of energy, and he walked so rapidly between the hospital and his laboratory on the seventh floor of the medical school that I, a fit young man that played squash twice a week, had difficulty keeping up with him. A tall, broad-shouldered, good-looking man with a full head of slightly grey-tinged black hair, often with a cigarette in his mouth, he also spoke rapidly, using terms and word sequences that I had difficulty understanding, prompting frequent visits to the medical library to look up unfamiliar words and ideas. My days were filled with ward rounds with the chief, pouring over large pages of data, modifying the doses of immunosuppressive drugs like cortisone, azathioprine, and cyclophosphamide based on daily blood tests and the patient's clinical condition. In addition, I saw potential kidney transplant patients in a weekly outpatient clinic, where I also met patients who had already received their transplants.

We never slept much because it was almost inevitable that we were called by the emergency room doctors in the middle of the night when they had a potential donor, usually from cadavers whose brains were dead but whose hearts stayed beating and where the kidneys functioned well. The process of selection of patients for transplantation in those days was primitive compared to the much more sophisticated process in modern times. My role was to take blood from the potential donor and walk it over to the lab at the medical school where a histocompatibility test was performed. Although the Major Histocompatibility Complex (MHC) of the mouse had been identified in the 1940s, the equivalent MHC in humans was still not completely known. Everything depended upon the red cell blood type and the Terasaki HLA test of the white cells from the donor to determine a potentially compatible recipient. Myburgh and the team looked at the results, and, from a potential list of kidney failure patients who might have been on dialysis for months, one was called to come in urgently to receive the new kidney.

A mere six years since he had done the first kidney transplant in South Africa, Myburgh was always emotionally charged, as if this were his very first case, and his anxiety made me nervous. Everything had to be just right, and his rapid talk seemed to take on even more urgency as we brought both donor and recipient to the operating rooms. The timing was critical since taking the kidney of the donor meant that the surgeon clamped the blood vessels supplying blood to the kidney, and that organ, like all other organs, could not survive too long without blood pumping through it. In the meantime, the anesthetized recipient in an adjacent room, an incision in the lower abdomen, was readied for the new kidney, carried sterile in a steel dish by a nurse from one operating room to another.

Even though I could see only the nurse's eyes, the rest of her face covered by a mask and surgical headgear, I imagined what she felt, praying and hoping that she would not trip and drop the precious organ on the floor. Everyone seemed to hold their breaths until the kidney was placed safely on the Mayo table, ready for Myburgh to sew it in place. He had been a world-class athlete, running four hundred-meter hurdles for South Africa, and his demeanor reminded me of the tension at a track event, the runners' muscles and minds waiting for the starter's pistol, adrenaline levels at a peak, hearts beating fast, breathing rapidly, eyes narrowed, focused on the track, taking off with hair trigger intensity, each athlete ready to be faster than anyone else.

I was tense as he lay the kidney down in the pelvis, making sure the donor kidney blood vessels and ureter were long enough, and identifying the recipient vessels where he was to do the anastomosis with Prolene suture. I had worked with vascular surgeons and had participated in many blood vessel connections, and everyone had their own technique of stitching. Myburgh had his own preferences, and I adapted to them quickly. The surgical technique had changed very little from the original pelvic operation. The kidney, cooled in an ice bath when removed from the donor and perfused with a special solution to remove all the donor blood, looked initially like a small, whitish-purple structure, about the size of my fist, and when the blood vessels were unclamped, the organ changing before our eyes, alive again with blood flowing in through the artery and out through the veins, and, quite quickly, drops of urine coming out of the ureter. The moment that happened, I could feel the tension in the room dissolve as everyone relaxed, and Bert seemed relieved.

Myburgh's animal lab on the seventh floor of the medical school was where we went every day after seeing human patients. His lab assistants had anesthetized two baboons from a cadre of about forty of these powerful creatures, sold to the medical school by farmers who laid traps for them on their farms where they would descend every night to steal pumpkins from the fields. Nobody had any qualms about experimenting on these animals, and I overcame my absolute horror when I first discovered how they were being used for experiments. Myburgh was the only person on earth doing transplants in baboons, and this gave him a unique leg-up on other transplant researchers who used dogs, pigs, and mice. The advantage of using baboons was that they were most like humans. He became well known around the world.

The ritual was the same every day. Myburgh's assistants removed the liver from the donor animal, and Myburgh put it into the other one after first removing the recipient liver. He connected vessels and the bile duct, five anastomoses that needed to be watertight and perfect, and once the clamps that blocked the flow of blood and bile were removed, with blood flowing through the new liver, the experiment was on to see how long the recipient lived, adding new methods or drugs to compare to the standard methods of immunosuppression. The animal was tranquilized every day to get blood for analysis, with massive amounts of data accumulating, like what happened to the human patients in the hospital. Myburgh had not yet done a liver transplant in human patients, but the objective was plainly apparent—that would come soon, during my time on the service.

The research scientist associated with the transplant program, Koos Smith, had a lot of equipment in his lab, and with my interest in research, I quickly persuaded him to let me do some studies on patients' white blood cells. I had become intrigued with a new assay, a chromium release assay, which had first been revealed in 1969, and it was a method to more accurately determine compatibility between donor and recipient lymphocytes, more accurate than relying on the Terasaki assay. It probably wasn't a practical way to determine ahead of time if a donor and recipient were compatible because each test took at least a day to complete, but I intended to see, in retrospect, how well it correlated with patients' outcomes. Little did I realize that the test would be my passport to my move to the States.

My rotation in Myburgh's transplant surgery unit gave me a front row seat to the immune system and lymph nodes involved in the immune responses to transplanted organs. The existence of two distinct but interacting lymphocyte subsets, one (T cells) derived from the thymus gland sitting in front of the heart in the upper chest and involved in cellular immunity, helping the other subset (B cells), derived from the bone marrow in producing antibody which was reported by Miller in 1961, when I was a first-year medical student. The importance of this observation came at a time when organ transplantation was beginning to take off in the 1960s, and no one really understood the role of lymphocytes in transplant organ rejection. It takes a while for new information to be truly incorporated into the understanding of its role in the physiology of the body.

How does serendipity work? How is it possible that an event occurs that completely alters the trajectory of one's life? I was due to complete my surgical training at the end of 1974, and there had been no question that I would stay in Johannesburg, perhaps as a lecturer in the surgery department where I would stay and become a transplant surgeon. One unplanned and unexpected event changed my plans, my accidental meeting with Arlene Levine, whom I had dated once when she was seventeen and I was aged nineteen and in medical school. She started medical school at Wits, married a young gastroenterologist, and moved to the States where he had a position at the University of Chicago. I had lost contact with her but recognized her picture and name on a hospital notice board, advertising that she would give a lecture on the chromium release assay at the South African Institute of Medical Research. Since I was doing the same assay in Smith's lab, and I was intrigued with her journey to the States and bursting with the intrigue about how she had ended up in the Virology Department at Rush Presbyterian St. Luke's Medical Center in Chicago, I went to listen to her talk.

I sat in the back of the auditorium listening to Arlene's lecture, impressed with her data and with her elegance. People gathered around her after she finished her talk, and I quietly waited to ask her some questions. She recognized me immediately.

"Hi, David. I thought I recognized you while I was talking. What are you doing now?"

We talked incessantly as I caught up with her life, shared mine, and we had lunch in the cafeteria. She had finished medical school at Northwestern University Medical Center in Chicago and started training in general surgery at Rush Presbyterian St. Luke's in Chicago, taking a year off to do the research that she had just presented. When I told her how I had taught myself to do the chromium release assay and how frustrating it was because the equipment I used was old and finicky, and the supplies difficult to come by, and there were no mentors available, she said: "Why don't you come and work with me in Chicago? I have a lab tech who works with me, and we've found something interesting in the blood of breast cancer patients that we're pursuing. You could spend a little time with us and see how we do the assay."

When I thought about it a little, and asked some questions, I decided that this would be an exciting addition to my planned visit to the International Congress of Immunology in Brighton, England, in July 1974. Living so far away from Europe and North America, naïve to international travel, I imagined that a flight across the Atlantic Ocean from London to Chicago would be easy. It would mean being away for at least six weeks from the last year of my surgical training, but I had enough vacation time banked to be able to do it.

My pursuit of interesting research in immunology was about to take a giant leap forward, changing my life completely.

CHAPTER 12

SEEING THE HIDDEN

Curiosity is the mainspring of a scientist's work. Experimentation is a restless endeavor to know. I had to know. Finding something new, something that I had hypothesized, after carrying out a tricky experiment gave me the exhilaration of discovery, a sense of reward, a satisfaction, a deeper feeling that Freud described as "oceanic." The feeling must somewhat mimic that of an Olympic swimmer winning the gold medal or a baseball slugger hitting the winning home run. This occasional feeling compensated for the disappointments and frustration of experiments that didn't work, and the realization that some of my favorite ideas were groundless.

During my journeys into the scientific world, I recognized that there were many different types of scientist that Peter Medawar called "collectors, classifiers, and those who need to compulsively tidy up." Some are detectives by nature, many are explorers, some are artisans, and some are artists. I had not yet reached my own zenith, and I still had a nagging feeling that I didn't have the smarts, or the research background, to be a good scientist. I had given myself an opportunity to find out by attending the Second International Congress of Immunology in Brighton in July 1974, just before spending time at Rush Presbyterian Medical Center in Chicago with Arlene.

My only previous experiences at large scientific meetings were workshops, symposia, or conferences in South Africa, and the presentations were filled with "artistic collectors," where clinicians, dressed in suits and ties, showed their great achievements in the form of pictures taken of patients, scientific tables describing patient demographics, perhaps a graph or two, or figures drawn by medical artists. Listening to world immunology experts in Brighton, very few wearing suits or ties, made me understand that the language of science as practiced by basic scientists in the rapidly advancing field of immunology was different from anything I had known previously.

The international community was agog with anticipation, and that year, there were several immunologists from major research universities around the world, some who had already been awarded Nobel Prizes, and some who were destined to win that prize or some other major international prize. Brunner and Cerottini, the two scientists whose work on the chromium release assay I had tried to do in Koos Smith's lab, gave talks that sparkled with facts and my surgical brain found difficulty in understanding. I was most intrigued with the recent discoveries of Zinkernagel and Doherty on an important way by which T-lymphocytes worked in transplant rejection. A newly identified cell, called "dendritic," was found to be important in the presentation of antigens to T-cells and, therefore, also vital in the transplant rejection phenomenon. My mind focused on everything to do with transplantation because I wanted to be a transplant surgeon.

The train journey from Brighton to London's Charing Cross station took an hour, and I traveled to see my brother, Alan, and his girlfriend, and to stay with his next-door neighbor, Avrion Mitchison, in his old Victorian-style house in Islington nearby. I took the Underground to the National Institute of Medical Research at Mill Hill to meet Professor Mitchison. Alan had arranged for me to meet Av in his office and he would take me to his house.

No one believed how I found Mitchison's office. Walking down long poorly marked corridors in the old building which had housed so many famous scientists, some of whom received Nobel Prizes for their work, I came across a disheveled, middle-aged guy in moth-eaten clothes, probably a janitor, and asked him where I could find professor Mitchison's office.

He pointed me in the right direction, and I thanked him and walked to the office which had Mitchison's name on it and, finding no one there, sat down and waited. Some minutes later, the same guy who had pointed me towards the office walked into the anteroom, introduced himself as "Av," and invited me into his clustered office, including some cages with mice that he proceeded to inject with a needle and syringe while talking to me.

Later that day he took me home to his house to meet Lorna, his wife, and his five children. The old Victorian-style house had five floors and an attic, which I accessed by a step ladder, dragging my suitcase precariously up through a hole in the ceiling to get to my guest bed. The Mitchisons hosted a party for several people that evening, including Peter Medawar, who had been Director of the NIMR until a few years before and a recipient of the Nobel Prize in Medicine and Physiology in 1962 for his groundbreaking research on immune tolerance. He wore a brace on his left leg and held his left arm in a sling, the result of a massive stroke a few years before, but his protégé, Liz Simpson, who ran his lab at NIMR until he left in 1972 to move to the Clinical Research Center at Northwick Park a few miles away, claimed that he knew more with 10 percent of his brain functioning than most people with 100 percent brain capacity. I hovered around the famous man, hoping to discuss some plans I had for doing immunology research in preparation for my planned career in transplantation. I had my chance and started telling him about "my" protein, but he interrupted me.

"I'm sure you have some interesting ideas, but I make it a rule to not discuss serious science at cocktail parties. Why don't you come and visit me tomorrow at Northwick Park and we can do a little experiment together?"

This was a phenomenal opportunity, and I took the underground train to the hospital where I found Medawar sitting behind his office desk. He encouraged me to tell him what hypothesis I planned to prove.

I told him about the protein that Klatzow and I had identified in the serum of terminal cancer patients, and in people with some chronic conditions, including patients in kidney failure. I had a portfolio of pictures of the polyacrylamide gel electrophoresis patterns that I had brought with me from Johannesburg.

"Do you know the name of the protein?" he asked.

"No, the only thing I can tell you is that it has a molecular weight of 48,000 and runs just in front of albumin in the electrophoresis."

"What do you think it does?"

Klatzow and I had speculated that this protein was immune suppressing in some way, but we had no real justification for that belief. We just knew that we should isolate the protein, do a few chemical experiments, and then mass-produce the chemical and use it the suppress the immune system in transplant patients.

Medawar listened carefully to my confident ramblings and looked at me and said: "Are you familiar with Thomas Hobbes?"

"Vaguely. Wasn't he an English writer?"

"A remarkably astute philosopher from the seventeenth century. I like to think of one of his quotes where he said that life is like a race, and the most important thing is to be in it, to be fully engaged, ambitious, and go-getting, and to improve the world. Do you think you can be fully into your project?"

"Absolutely!"

"Before I talk to you about what experiments you would plan for this mysterious protein, I would like you to do a quick lab experiment right now."

"Right now?"

"Yes. Would you be willing to spend a few hours doing a little lab work for me?"

"I guess so. What did you have in mind?"

"Write this down, and I'll have one of my lab techs show you where the supplies are."

He described what he wanted me to do, and a little bewildered, I asked him how that would be important to do before he could advise me about the series of experiments I was planning to do upon my return to South Africa.

"It's quick and easy and will give me an idea about whether you understand small details in the lab."

The "experiment" took me about two hours. I thought it was stupid, but I did it anyway because I needed to get the advice of this important man of science.

I took one hundred small glass tubes, labeled them with a pen, weighed each one, wrote down the weight on a lab book page, put each tube in order in a wooden rack, pipetted one hundred microliters of distilled water into each tube, weighed them, recorded the weights in the lab book, subtracted the initial weight, recorded the weight of the water I had pipetted and presented the sheet to Medawar. It was the sort of lab practice that one would do in a high school science lab.

"What are your conclusions?" he asked.

"It looks like the volume of water that I pipetted into each tube varied somewhat, some being a little more than one hundred microliters, some a little less."

"What do you think that means?"

"I guess it means that my pipetting skills are a little rusty and not absolutely perfect and reproducible. But I'm sure I can improve and get exactly the right volume pipetted every time."

"Partly true, yes. But no one is ever perfect in the lab. The message for you is that you have to accept that experiments in immunology will vary depending upon many variables, and one of those is the way that you yourself do the measuring. That is why you need to repeat experiments. Each observation point should be done in triplicate and then repeat the experiments on separate days. I urge you to think about this because it is common for clinicians like you to observe one time and to accept that is the conclusion."

This did not surprise me because I had experienced something similar in my home photographic lab, my sickle cell thalassemia project, the tooth study with Tobias, the experiments with the chromium release assay that that I had done in Koos Smith's lab, and with Klatzow's polyacrylamide gel serum study. I recognized the truth of his observations about clinicians doing clinical studies.

Medawar's parting words that day were sharp and insightful.

"If you want to be successful in research, you should do something that is not only uniquely new but also extremely important. A scientist who studies dull or piffling problems finds dull or piffling answers. When you have a 'brainwave,' an idea you think is unique, spend time in the library and make sure it is new. Quite often you will find someone else has studied the problem in depth. If it is new, it is truly unseen, and you aim to uncover the unseen by being the first to see it in your mind. That is not enough. You must design experiments and controls that lead to results that are incontrovertible. Newton and Einstein's findings are still valuable now even if they have been advanced by others. Whatever you discover must be valuable anywhere and anytime on Earth, but also everywhere in the universe."

There is something breathtaking about the minds of people like Medawar and Mitchison, a freshness, almost like a cleansing wind blowing across the Sahara Desert, because they think deeply on their feet and come up with ideas. Their scientific minds questioned everything around them and within their sphere of intelligence. I realized that I, like many of the sophisticated lab scientists I had met in Britain, sought answers ranging from what exists at the edge of our universe to the reasons behind why we they even exist, and explanations for everything and anything. They appeared to have four personality characteristics in common—curiosity, an open mind, skepticism, and humility, finding happiness in breaking things down to their elementary parts, and seeing the beauty and feeling the awe of the minutest of entities. I noticed them constantly seeking to reason out everything they were exposed to, looking to find a story behind the events that led to an observation and conclusion. I watched Mitchison dissect everyday life and find more meaning in the most trivial of things. His razor-sharp mind allowed him to filter everything through the framework of knowledge he had gained, and his dry British wit made him appear indifferent to the opinion of cynics.

After my short time in England, exposed to basic scientists, I left for Chicago to work with Arlene, armed with fresh ideas about how to move forward with my own research. I was ready to scrutinize any facts presented before me and only accept those after careful thought, accept the truth, however bitter it might be, and not conceal it with more acceptable but inaccurate explanations, and concentrate on finding an underlying pattern or relations which might bind the parts of the whole together.

Chapter 13

Eyes Wide Open

In this world of great diversity, my visit to Chicago in 1974 to spend a few weeks with Arlene in her lab in the Virology Department at Rush Presbyterian St Luke's Medical Center provided me an opening into an environment I had not anticipated or even requested. In retrospect, it is almost as though I had a guardian angel leading me confidently from one steppingstone to another, without feeling any uncertainty. Like Thomas Cole's series of paintings, *Voyages of Life*, a series of four paintings representing an allegory of the four stages of human life, depicting a voyager who travels in a boat on a river through the mid-nineteenth century American wilderness accompanied by a guardian angel, I saw a shining castle in the sky, the lab time where I would bring my newfound understanding of the scientific mindset and learn something important and new.

Naïve to the exigencies of urban Chicago life, I arrived by cab at the hospital with my suitcase, met Arlene and the lab staff, and prepared to walk the three blocks to the University of Illinois Medical Dormitory where I was to stay, when a policeman at the hospital entrance stopped me and asked where I was headed. When I told him who I was and where I was going, he offered to take me in his patrol car.

"It's only three blocks," I said. "I'll be fine, thanks,"

"This is a rough neighborhood, Doc. I'll take you. Hop in."

That was the beginning of a wonderful awakening to American friendliness, contradicting the stories I had heard of "the rudeness" I was sure to encounter, the so-called "dirty American" that Europeans publicize, during my first visit to North America.

Arlene and I worked side by side for a week in the lab before she introduced me to the chairman of the Department of Virology, Friedrich Dienhardt, a distinguished leader of great vision, achievement, and purpose, internationally renowned for his studies in infectious diseases, cancer, and in primates, particularly in identifying a virus that caused hepatitis in marmosets. He knew Peter Medawar, and when I discussed my visit to his lab at Northwick Park, he invited me to tell him more about my plans over dinner at his house.

Fritz, as he insisted I call him with his delightful German accent, and his English-born wife, Joan, an immunologist herself, asked me after dinner what I planned for my future.

"I have a position back home in the department of surgery. I want to be a transplant surgeon."

"Is there a training program, a fellowship, in transplant surgery in South Africa?" Fritz asked.

"No, there isn't."

"It's interesting that you should want to do basic research in the immunology of transplantation," said Joan, "but I wonder if you wouldn't be better off looking for a sophisticated group of immunologists in the States or in Europe to do that before you concentrate on transplant surgery. You would put yourself in a great position to lead the field with that kind of background."

"Do you have a group here in Chicago that I can talk to about that?" I asked.

Fritz suggested I start by introducing myself to the chief of surgical oncology at the University of Illinois Medical Center a few blocks down the street.

"I know Das Gupta, and he is a surgeon doing lab research so, even though it is not transplantation, the immunology currently developing in both the fields of oncology and transplantation are somewhat similar. My secretary can help you. I'll also make a few calls around the country, speak to my colleagues, and we can set up a series of interviews for you."

Das Gupta reminded me of my surgical colleagues back in Johannesburg in the manner of his militaristic-style offer that would guarantee a position in his division of surgical oncology for only six months, during which time I would be expected to produce at least one scientific paper. I felt that would be impossible for a foreign doctor to accomplish considering my need to adapt first to the culture of America and Chicago. I also wasn't really interested in surgical oncology. Besides, there were other places and people to visit.

Traveling around the United States for two weeks, visiting lab scientists in Minneapolis, Denver, San Francisco, Los Angeles, Baltimore, New York, Bethesda, and Boston opened my eyes to the exciting new world of immunologic research in North America. One of my first interviews was with Ronald Herberman, Chief of the Laboratory of Immunodiagnosis at the National Cancer Institute in Bethesda, who suggested I might benefit most from the environment of international scientists at NIH studying the "new immunology." While visiting him in Building 10 as part of the world's largest clinical research center, I took the opportunity to visit Stephen Rosenberg, newly appointed chief of the surgery branch and head of the tumor immunology section, who had begun to recruit young scientists and fellows. He asked if I would be interested in spending two years with him. We set the wheels in motion, a process that required me to either be a citizen, which I was not, or to get a green card, a way to become a citizen in five or six years. Neither of us had the knowledge or expertise to work out the bureaucracy to make this happen, and I reluctantly let that fellowship opportunity disappear. As my career blossomed in other areas, I watched Rosenberg pioneer the development of effective immunotherapies and gene therapies for patients with advanced cancers. His studies of the adoptive transfer of genetically modified lymphocytes have resulted in the regression of metastatic cancer in patients with melanoma, sarcomas, and lymphomas. In retrospect, my contributions to sentinel node biopsy would probably not have materialized if I had stayed with Rosenberg.

One visits a famous university or other type of medical center as a foreigner, armed with one's own cultural background, knowing American culture only from watching movies or studying American literature, missing the true reality by not having lived in it. In August 1974, the frenetic customs of the east coast, coupled with the uncomfortable heat and humidity, so different from the character of life and climate in Johannesburg, was enough to discourage me from immediately taking up the offers for fellowship training from the various medical centers in Boston, New York, and Baltimore. I just didn't feel comfortable in those places. In contrast, in Los Angeles when I visited the Department of Immunology and Microbiology at UCLA in Westwood, the first thing that struck me was how pleasant it was to walk around the beautiful campus in brilliant sunshine and low humidity. There, I felt at home.

That was when I first met John L Fahey, chairman of the Department of Immunology and Microbiology at UCLA, one of the founding fathers of the field of clinical immunology, who had discovered Immunoglobulin D (IgD) while at NIH and delineated other classes of immunoglobulins. Later, also famous for building research capacity for HIV/AIDS in developing countries, one of his major contributions in the fight against AIDS was his research in the interaction of the immune system and the nervous system, pointing out the complexity of the disease.

Something about the friendly way I was introduced to the faculty at UCLA might have been because Fritz knew Fahey and introduced me as "someone who spent time with Peter Medawar," even though it had only been one day. Nobody needed to know that. I felt like a celebrity walking through the fourth floor of the UCLA medical center with gleaming labs filled with supplies and equipment, most of the labs looking out of large windows at sun-filled gardens and clean-looking campus buildings. Meeting graduate students and their professors gave me a sense of the depth of intellect in the department, and Ben Bonavida, a young assistant professor in the department, took me to lunch at The Bomb Shelter, one of many outdoor restaurants on the campus that helped the students take advantage of the beautiful weather.

I was a little surprised by one faculty member, W H Hildeman, who tried hard to dissuade me from coming to UCLA, telling me to check out the medical library, one of the largest in the world, where I would find many books with pages torn out by students. I quickly discovered that he was a disgruntled professor, aspiring chairman of the medical immunology department before the committee selected Fahey, who had been caught in the move to modernize immunology, a difficult enough task for those of us eager young trainees but made more difficult for him because his expertise was in marine biology and immunology, not exactly directly related to the rapidly changing understanding of human and animal immunology. I heard from students that he and Fahey had competed for the chairmanship, partly explaining why he may have tried to derail any of Fahey's recruitment efforts. I came to an understanding with Fahey that I would return the following year to his department after I finished my surgical training.

Back with Arlene in Chicago, I discovered her secret. She had taken two years away from surgical training at Rush to do research on the immunology of breast cancer because she herself had the disease. She had developed breast cancer at age twenty-eight and had a radical mastectomy followed by chemotherapy and radiation. She kept this information private, but I knew something had happened to her right arm because I noticed she had a lymphedema sleeve and her right hand was swollen.

Lymphedema, or swelling of a part of the body because of blocked flow of lymph, was a condition that I had seen during my surgical training, and I knew a chronic swollen arm was possible after mastectomy. Seeing Arlene connect her arm to an external pump at night in her apartment overlooking Lake Michigan, after she confided her problem to me, was more real than seeing my patients in the Johannesburg General Hospital clinic. Comparing her shirt and blouse sleeves, I noticed the difference in size of the left versus the right. She had all her lymph nodes from the right armpit removed, an operation I had done myself, and I always made my patients aware that they could get lymphedema with that procedure. But, before I knew of Arlene's plight, I always thought it was a minor annoyance, telling myself and my patients it was a small price to pay for the possibility of cure from the breast cancer. Now I became aware that it was not a minor problem, and Arlene talked to me about her constant regret that she had the operation, especially now that she had metastases in her right lung and the uncomfortable breast and armpit surgery had not cured her. She believed that some women with early breast cancer might be cured with smaller operations.

"What sort of operation are you talking about?" I asked.

"I'm not sure that anyone has tried to take less lymph nodes to avoid lymphedema. This is something I'd like to work on someday."

"If you took less lymph nodes during surgery, you might miss taking the ones where the breast cancer has spread. If you left behind lymph nodes with tumor already in them, and you didn't know that, you would pretty much condemn your patients to recurrence with lethal spread to other organs. You can avoid that by taking all the lymph nodes. That's why we do that operation," I said.

"What if we could identify the lymph nodes with tumor and we took only those out?" she asked.

"I don't believe there is a way to do that, do you?"

"No, but there must be a way to find those nodes during surgery. Let's think about that a little over the next few days."

I loved the way she thought about problems, talked about ways to overcome them, and then proposed a solution. I worked with her in the lab, watching her do chromium release assays with Ken, her lab assistant, and change direction if that's what was required, or tenaciously keep repeating the same experiments repeatedly to verify results. She had found a specific type of lymphoid cell in the peripheral blood of her breast cancer population, one which seemed to correlate with the stage of the disease. Three years later, after she had spent research time at the National Cancer Institute and identified a third type of lymphocyte in human blood, which came to be known as a natural killer cell, Ron Herberman, the director of the lab, wrote a beautiful obituary to her in the Journal of the National Cancer Institute, acknowledging her unique contribution to tumor immunology.

Because of Arlene, I came to the USA, to Fahey's department at UCLA, intent on studying tumor immunology, remembering not only her thorough research habits, but also the probing mind that asked important questions. She had planted in me a question about how to overcome and prevent lymphedema in breast cancer, a question that haunted me for years, and that eventually helped address one of the most important changes in the surgical treatment of breast cancer, melanoma, and many other cancers. How sad she didn't live to see those dramatic advances.

Chapter 14

Westwood Bound

Arriving in Westwood, a suburb of Los Angeles, I had my work cut out to find a place to stay and a car to get me to the UCLA campus, a bank to do my financial business, and get used to every cultural detail that the average American learns over a life time of growing up. I might have been smart and have completed a surgical training program after medical school, but I had to learn how to drive on the right side of the road, having driven for twelve years on the left side of the road in cars with a steering wheel on the right side. That was only one of my many challenges in learning how to live in America.

My first visit to the Bel Aire supermarket near the UCLA campus was as bewildering as my first effort at driving my new car on the right side of the road. I couldn't decide which of the myriad bottles and containers in the milk stand was really "milk." Back home in South Africa, milk came in a bottle, delivered in the early hours of the morning by the milkman. Here I stood in front of different containers, all labeled "milk," some with calcium, some with vitamin D, some "whole," some "half and half," some "two percent," some with chocolate added. A woman, guiding her cart expertly past the milk stand, and in a hurry, looked impatiently at me when I asked her which one of these many options was milk.

"Can't you read?"

And off she went.

This was to be the pattern of my adaptation to my new home in Santa Monica, an apartment which had additional bamboozling aspects that most foreigners could not understand. First and last month's rent plus damage insurance? In Johannesburg, one signed a lease contract and paid the landlord every month. Paying extra for a parking spot? I was used to that being included back home. Clauses that suggested the landlord could raise the rent at any time? In Johannesburg, the rents were rarely raised in the first five years of occupancy.

My days in the Department of Immunology and Microbiology with John Fahey were even more confusing. While skilled at surgical procedures, I quickly grew frustrated at the lab procedures, assigned to a group of people in a new division, Cancer Immunodiagnosis, with assays done on the blood of cancer patients and controls as part of a new effort to prove that immunosuppression in cancer patients could be measured.

Medawar's advice soon loomed large in my psyche when I failed to see any of the assays showing evidence of change in patients' blood tests that proved they were immunosuppressed: "*If you want to be successful in research, you should do something that is not only uniquely new but also extremely important. A graduate student who studies dull or piffling problems finds dull or piffling answers.*"

When I started my research fellowship, immunosuppression in cancer was a largely unproven concept on everyone's mind. I had joined the "immunosuppression" lab at UCLA thinking that it was important enough for me to satisfy Medawar's advice. But now, six months later, I sensed I was wasting my time. I discussed this with Fahey, and he was open to giving me an opportunity to do something else.

After reading extensively and attending an "Immunology 101" class with freshmen undergraduates, I told Fahey I wanted to continue looking at the protein I had found with Klatzow in Johannesburg and to work on peripheral blood monocytes, a cell type that nobody thought important in immunology but which I believed would prove valuable. Fahey was skeptical, since everyone in his department worked on lymphocytes in one way or another, and monocytes did not seem important in immunosuppression in cancer patients, a concept that he and others felt was the future of immunology in cancer.

We had to identify tests that would be valuable in the clinic and prove an idea that had only vague supporting evidence. He was not supportive of me working on the protein.

My friend Ian Drew, who had traveled with me from Johannesburg, had a position in Paul Terasaki's lab in Westwood where he was involved with projects related to transplantation in humans, and he introduced me to his chief who assigned to me Ahmed, a young biochemist, to work on the protein project while I worked on monocytes. Both projects tended to satisfy Medawar's advice of doing something important, and I became excited again, believing that I could find something unique and new.

The incongruity associated with doing lab research by a fully trained surgeon played out in my approach to doing these two projects. With Fahey's blessing, I hired Peter, who had recently graduated with a degree in biology from UC Irvine, to do the lab work while I devoted my time to getting blood from patients and control normal people, and designing experiments, and we developed a way to separate monocytes from the peripheral blood, a way that helped us evaluate a unique ability of these cells to migrate towards a chemical stimulus, known as chemotaxis, a way for them to exert their biological activities, including moving from blood into the tissues where they changed into macrophages.

Working on monocytes and macrophages in an immunology department in the 1970s was like David facing Goliath. I liked the idea of studying these cells because they were active eaters, also called "phagocytes" (phage being derived from the Greek word for "eat") of dead cells, microbes, cancer cells, and any substance that is foreign. The importance of macrophages in inflammation and the importance of cells in immunity had been defined by Metchnikoff in Russia at least seventy-five years before my arrival in Los Angeles, but for some reason, that remains unclear to me to this day, my immunology colleagues at the time did not think these cells were part of the immune system. Years later, these cells were found to play a critical role in nonspecific defense (innate immunity) and also to help initiate specific defense mechanisms (adaptive immunity) by recruiting other immune cells such as lymphocytes.

The protein electrophoresis project in Terasaki's lab proved to be quite interesting as well, and it meant that I walked from the UCLA hospital, about four blocks, to the other lab to look at results with Ahmed, who, by doing basic chemistry, isolated the protein and helped me to prove that it was indeed immunosuppressive in that it inhibited the growth and multiplying of lymphocytes in test tube incubation studies.

Doing research was fun, but it hardly paid the bills nor was I in a position to compete for any permanent position as a lab scientist, and I wanted to get back into taking care of patients. It seemed that I had to do an internship in an approved program in California and pass an examination to get a license to practice medicine. There was no reciprocity for my years of surgical training in South Africa, but Fahey worked out a deal with the chairman of the Internal Medicine Department that I could be registered as an intern at UCLA while working part time in the newly formed Clinical Immunology and Allergy (CIA) program, designed to attend to the needs of patients with immune system abnormalities, either acquired from some disease, such as lupus, or cancer or from drugs used in transplantation or inherited. I spent a year in the CIA seeing patients with all kinds of immune dysfunction, including a new disease that seemed to destroy the immune systems of homosexual men, later shown to be HIV/AIDS. We didn't realize the importance of this devastating disease because it only started to appear in a very small number of patients in the 1970s.

The hospital cafeteria at UCLA hospital buzzed with people at lunch, and I had an opportunity to talk to surgeons in various programs. I had been away from surgeons for quite a while and had not done any surgery myself while working in the lab with technicians, graduate students, and an immunology faculty that was mostly comprised of basic scientists with PhDs. The transplant surgeons always seemed over-tired, and remembering my own time on the transplant service in Johannesburg, I could understand that they spent many nights operating and without sleep.

Another group of surgeons caught my eye, and I came to understand that they were surgical oncologists, specialists in the surgical management of cancers. They seemed less stressed because most of their surgeries were elective, done during daytime hours and only rarely at night. They also seemed friendly and somehow better groomed and dressed than the other surgeons, and I introduced myself and discovered that their chief was a man by the name of Donald L Morton who ran the division of surgical oncology at UCLA, a division that had been newly formed in 1971 when William Longmire, famed chairman of the UCLA Surgery Department, created the position and invited Morton, then chief of Tumor Immunology in the Surgery Branch at the National Cancer Institute, to be the chief.

In May 1977, close to the end of my immunology fellowship and with no position ahead of me in July, I experienced one of those almost unbelievable miracles that, looking back, had to have been because my guardian angel was looking out for me. A surgical oncology trainee greeted me at the cafeteria at lunch time and asked if I had heard the news that one of the surgical oncology fellows due to start in July had pulled out. That meant there was a position available, and he wondered if I was interested. He gave me Morton's telephone number, and I called immediately.

Morton's secretary promptly put him on the telephone, and he asked me if I had a California physician license.

"Yes," I said.

"Come and see me so we can talk about this position. My office is in the Security Pacific Bank Building on Le Conte Avenue."

My first meeting with Morton gave me a sense of how lucky I would be to work with him. A large man with a surprisingly high-pitched voice, he asked me what I had been doing in the immunology lab and told me I would fit perfectly with his lab scientists and suggested I meet them so I could decide what project to do when I started in July.

I had lived briefly in a world of basic scientists and learned that science can mean different things to different people. I had a dream that explained why surgeons think it a waste of time to do basic science research and why basic scientists think that surgeons trying to do basic science research should stick to being in the operating room. I created a cartoon, based on a story of bodies floating down a river. On the river bank were four different types of surgical scientists: the first, equivalent to the surgical types I had known, a man in a white coat, kneeling trying to remove as many of the bodies as he could, and reporting how many of these people he had saved and how many had been lost. This would be like the surgeons who did an operation well and created papers based on their surgical excellence. The next type, also reminiscent of surgeons doing research, was a man in a suit with a notebook, counting the bodies floating by. When asked what he was doing, he replied: "I'm making a database, and when I have enough cases, I'll analyze the data and write a few papers." I thought that type of research would interest a certain type of person who wasn't familiar or interested in hypothesis-driven science. The third type of person in my cartoon is not even looking at the river and represents the basic scientist who is thinking about all sorts of basic science questions and coming up with experiments that will do nothing to save the people floating down the river but may point to issues to be seen in the future, such as Einstein's theories in relativity and how they were essential to the discovery of space flight and lasers and the digital age. I had tried that in the immunology department and realized that was not for me. I aspired to be the fourth type of surgical-scientist, the man who had a pair of binoculars trained up stream and, when asked what he was doing, said: "I want to find out what's happening up stream, so I can work out how to prevent this tragedy that is happening."

My guardian angel was about to introduce me to my future, where I would look upstream for causes and mechanisms in tumor biology, looking for inexhaustible problems that needed fixing.

Chapter 15

Lymphedema

I was indirectly introduced to Don through his fellows in the UCLA cafeteria when I was a fellow in Immunology in John Fahey's department. I heard stories over lunch of his recruitment to UCLA in 1971 when he assumed the role of professor and chief of the Division of Surgical Oncology within the department of general surgery where he had a unique mentoring quality that allowed him to pass on his experience and wisdom to young clinicians and basic science faculty, an important attribute that I longed to experience. He had received long-term NCI funding to conduct phase I, II, and III trials of non-specific active immunotherapy, including intralesional Bacillus Calmette-Guerin (BCG) for melanoma, development of monoclonal antibodies, biologic modifiers, and therapeutic melanoma vaccines, and had developed a world-renowned, research-oriented cancer treatment center, one of the largest melanoma referral centers in the country, and had become "surgical oncologist to the Hollywood elite."

I joined his training program in 1977 as the fifteenth surgical oncology fellow under his tutelage. The surgical oncology clinic on the fourth floor of the Security Pacific Bank Building on the corner of Le Conte Avenue and Westwood Boulevard, at the entrance to the UCLA campus and a block away from the UCLA Medical Center, looked like a plush private physicians' office, luxuriously furnished, a giant fish tank in the middle of the waiting room, expensive-looking artworks on the walls, and the entrance invitingly manned by friendly well-dressed staff. On my first day as a surgical oncology fellow, I was escorted to my new office, shared with Charles Callery, a UCLA surgical resident taking two years out of his general surgery training to do research with Morton. After a brief guided walkthrough of the clinic, where I was introduced to clinical and research nurses, medical assistants, and some of the junior faculty, I was ushered into Morton's office.

There he was, my new chief with a crew-cut hairstyle, sitting comfortably behind a large mahogany desk, not looking at all like a poor boy from West Virginia. It could have been a little intimidating for a young trainee to sit in the luxurious office of a living legend, and I didn't know what to expect. Most surgical trainees in all the academic surgery departments I had visited in four countries seemed intensely cautious of their chiefs, always alert to critical comments, fearful of being blamed for complications after operations on patients, and potentially at risk of career-ending terminations. I needn't have worried. I soon realized that he wanted me to feel right at home and to succeed.

"Welcome, David," he said, smiling broadly.

He seemed genuinely interested in my past research and asked me to explain some of the experiments I had done in Immunology at UCLA during my two years in Fahey's department as he asked me detailed questions.

"We have a strong research component in the Division of Surgical Oncology, and I would like you to look through this portfolio of fifty research projects that might interest you. Once you've looked through them, please connect with the people that run those projects and decide which lab you'd like to join to do your research. Since you're on an NIH training grant, you will have some funds devoted to supplies, and if there is equipment you need, please speak to Sid Golub or Reiko Irie, and we'll see if we can accommodate your needs. We all meet once a week on Thursday morning to discuss our research. As far as your clinical responsibilities are concerned, you'll be working mostly with me on Wednesdays in the clinic, and we'll talk in more detail next week about our comprehensive note-taking on patients."

Piggybacking on existing research projects was, and still is, standard for young trainees, but I had ideas of my own, and I was more advanced both clinically and in immunology research than the other fellows who were mostly young surgeons-in-training from around the country. I still had incomplete projects from my fellowship in immunology with Fahey that I wanted to complete, especially my study of cancer patients exhibiting an immunosuppressive protein that I had first discovered with David Klatzow in Johannesburg and just recently continued developing with Ahmed in Teresaki's department. Morton supported my continued research on this protein and suggested I work with Rishab Gupta in his lab at the Veteran's Hospital in Northridge, fifteen miles from the UCLA campus. Rishab had some expertise in protein chemistry and was part of Morton's surgical oncology "empire," which included two VA hospitals and the UCLA Medical Center.

Over the next week or so, I became aware of the archival specimen resource that Morton had started soon after coming to Los Angeles. This was an outstanding collection of serum and cells from every patient treated in the Division of Surgical Oncology. A team of people assigned to the task collected blood from every patient, separated the serum and cells, and froze each specimen to minus 196 degrees Celsius, stored at that temperature in liquid nitrogen freezers. The repository of specimens was so valuable that the team was on call day and night in case there was an electrical failure or any other disaster since unintentional thawing of the specimens would result in loss of precious research opportunities. The priceless value of these specimens, coupled with clinical information on every patient, was strongly endorsed by reviewing study sections at the National Cancer Institute that repeatedly funded Morton's program projects so that he was eventually known for a record-setting level of multiple continuous NIH-funded program projects, producing countless translational studies and scientific publications. I realized how important this asset was to my own research since I was eligible, as a member of the Division, to obtain samples and to do research that few other researchers could do.

My Wednesday clinics with Morton gave me a ringside seat to his clinical and research wisdom and his dedication to patient care. He sincerely believed that there was a genetic link between kindness and the likelihood of getting cancer because he had a deep emotional connection with patients he saw with me in the clinic and thought they were "the nicest people in the world." Patients came from all over the world to see him, and he treated them all with respect and empathy. My role was to "work up" the patient, take a detailed clinical history, do an examination, and then call him in. We discussed the patients in his office, sometimes over lunch, and planned a course of action. At the end of the day, the entire Division of Surgical Oncology, with physicians from Radiation and Medical Oncology, met in the library to discuss all the new patients and some follow-up cases.

It was during one of the Multidisciplinary Cancer Conferences that I first became aware of a new scan that Morton introduced in patients with melanoma. Melanoma, a potentially highly lethal form of skin cancer, was usually treated with surgical excision of the pigmented tumor. In many patients, that treatment was enough to cure almost 100 percent of people with the disease. However, some patients needed to have their lymph nodes removed as well. Patients with arm melanomas would have their armpit lymph nodes removed, an operation called a complete axillary lymphadenectomy. Patients with leg melanomas would sometimes have their groin lymph nodes removed, an operation called radical inguino-pelvic lymphadenectomy. The rationale for these lymphadenectomies was based upon the belief that the melanoma could spread first to the nearest lymph nodes, the regional lymph nodes, before spreading to internal organs in the body, such as the liver, lungs, brain, or bone. Surgeons believed that surgical removal of lymph nodes containing melanoma metastases could cure a substantial number of patients at a time when there were no other treatments available. Patients with melanomas of the skin of the chest, abdomen, buttocks, perineum, and the head and neck presented a problem that differed from melanomas of the limbs where the flow of lymph had to go through the groin or armpit on the same side. A melanoma of the skin of the left side of the abdomen could spread through the lymphatics to the lymph nodes in the groin, armpit, or even the neck, and even to the opposite side of the patient's body. Morton's scan entailed injecting radioactive colloidal gold into the skin around the melanoma and taking a picture of the patient with a gamma camera about an hour later. The lymph nodes lit up only in the site where the melanoma might spread in the neck, armpit, or groin and would guide the surgeon as to which lymph nodes to remove.

Intrigued with the radioactive lymph node scan, I began to think about the conversation I had with Arlene in Chicago and about all those patients I had already seen with chronic limb swelling after lymphadenectomies. What if we could find the one or two lymph nodes identified with the scan in the operating room? Surely that would save many patients from having all their nodes removed. Maybe we didn't have to remove all the nodes even in those seventeen percent of melanoma patients with lymph node metastases. But there was no technology at the time that would enable us to find those radioactive nodes, and I reluctantly put that idea in the vault of my memory, not completely forgotten, and re-opened about nine years later. While I was with Morton, seeing about a thousand new melanoma patients per year, he was able to report on the value of the scan in 1,415 patients in a paper published in 1978.

Emotions can be raw for both people the first time a surgeon confronts a patient with a potentially lethal cancer recurrence. I had learned to deal privately with those feelings, and years of dealing with dying patients taught me to perpetuate my own emotional blocking techniques so I could distance myself from human tragedies of patients and their grieving families.

But Helen changed all that.

One of my first patients with Morton, I reviewed her surgery for a back melanoma done by the chief two years before the current visit before entering the examining room in the clinic to meet her. I introduced myself to Helen and her husband, who anxiously clutched each other, tears streaming down their cheeks.

"What's happening? I looked at your notes from the last visit and everything seemed okay apart from your swollen arm."

"I'm worried about this lump," she said, pointing with her right hand to the left upper back.

I examined her and noted her swollen left arm and a small subcutaneous lump next to the scar over her scapula. The swollen arm reminded me of many other patients I had seen with lymphedema following removal of multiple lymph nodes in the armpit.

"Is that lump new?" I asked.

She nodded, exploring my face for signs of optimism. I tried adopting my usual professional stance, expecting this would protect me from the pain of having to tell her we needed to do a biopsy, to remove the lump in the small operating room next door. I'm not a good poker player, and try as I might, I could not hide from her probing eyes.

This is the professional way to do these things. Just keep calm, stay supportive, carefully explain what needs to be done, I told myself. *Don't let on how certain you are that this is a local recurrence of her melanoma.*

We met again the following week when I had the result of her biopsy. Recurrent melanoma, subcutaneous. The likelihood of spread to other parts of her body was high, and we soon discovered it had already spread to her lungs. In 1977 there was no good treatment for stage four melanoma, and I was not sure how to tell her this in a kind way.

"I'm going to refer you to another doctor to take care of you," I said.

But Helen protested.

"They told me that you're my doctor," she said. "I trust you and Doctor Morton. I don't want another doctor. Besides that, I need help with my swollen arm, and this is the best clinic for that. I need you to give me new elastic stocking for my arm, and I may need a pump at night."

I relented, weighing her needs and the focus she had on her lymphedema.

"Okay. Let's see what Doctor Morton says."

Morton was visibly disturbed by Helen's recurrence, but his eternal optimism emerged quickly as he told her that we had treatment that might help her.

The medical profession indulges in technological wizardry and super-specialized body mechanics, and I was proud of my own achievements, learning how to do all manner of surgical oncology operations with Morton and his faculty, some of the best in the world. In my monumental struggle to prolong life, I had paid little attention to the quality of the patient's remaining days, relying on others to take care of psychological, spiritual, and mechanical needs. Helen's needs showed me how I had lost the holistic point of view which was characteristic of a former era when there was usually no other way to help patients than to show empathy and compassion.

Helen's physical needs were evident because I spent a lot of time with her, both in the clinic and when she was admitted to the hospital. Just like my experience with other lymphedema patients, I saw how difficult it was to adapt to a swollen arm, and I realized that simple daily activities of living were adversely affected because of the lymphedema; I saw Helen's struggle with clothes, elastic arm stockings, uncomfortable at best, hot and horrible in the heat of summer, and mechanical pumps. This got me thinking again about whether removing all her armpit lymph nodes had been appropriate treatment, especially since none of the removed lymph nodes had contained any metastatic tumor. The lymphadenectomy had not helped her, and now she was dying of the disease anyway while suffering with the swollen arm.

Morton's clinical practice for melanoma and breast cancer followed accepted guidelines prevalent in North America at the time and included removing all the lymph nodes in the armpit, or the neck, or the groin, depending upon where the melanoma was found. Swollen upper or lower limbs followed in some patients and produced a change in lifestyle, and often in patients who might have survived as well without having the lymph nodes removed. When I questioned the practice, having been trained in South Africa to remove all the lymph nodes only when there was clear-cut melanoma clinically apparent spread to the nodes, Morton smiled and told me that waiting for patients to develop lymph node metastasis would condemn many to a potentially preventable, untreatable further spread to internal organs with a higher likelihood of dying compared to patients who had those nodes removed when the amount of tumor in the node was tiny.

"It seems that some patients without tumor in the lymph nodes, who might have avoided having them removed altogether, have developed chronic, incurable limb swelling, and they constitute most people with this disease," I said.

"You may be right about patients like Helen who clearly didn't benefit from having all her nodes removed. She was unlucky to develop significant lymphedema, but we don't see that many patients with chronic lymphedema after lymphadenectomy, David," said Morton.

"Maybe we don't see them because they don't come back to us and see other doctors."

"We keep careful records of patients even when they don't come back to us," said Morton. "We send reminders to referring doctors that takes care of the issue."

That didn't satisfy me because I wasn't certain that notes obtained from other doctors seeing Morton's patients would accurately document the existence of lymphedema, especially if those doctors were not specifically looking for that complication of the procedure.

"Maybe we can develop a test that doesn't require removing all the nodes to find out which patients might benefit from lymphadenectomy."

He smiled and nodded his head, but I wasn't sure he agreed. We didn't talk about that until many years later, when he and I had begun to study the issue and when techniques developed in mice could be translated into a major advance in the management of melanoma and the prevention of lymphedema.

Chapter 16

Principal Investigator

Events sometimes develop by chance, and a series of happy occasions may be beneficial in many ways to many people. My lab on the fourth floor of the Education and Research Building at Henry Ford Hospital in Detroit led to a series of personal and social processes that motivated chance experiments and discoveries that helped change the way surgeons around the world treat melanoma and breast cancer.

I brought with me from my meanderings around the world of medicine and science a theoretical framework for discovering new information, formulating questions, and a conscious and unconscious immersion in the lymphatic system. Primed by my practical surgical training in the removal of lymph nodes and my intense exposure to scientists studying basic tumor immunology at UCLA, I focused on designing an experimental program by concentrating my initial efforts on embedding my mind in the literature of mechanisms of lymph node metastasis, immune responses to tumors, and the biology of human tumors. Given my exposure to the lymphatic system initially during childhood, and repeated serendipitous later exposure to this mysterious and largely unseen system, I found myself eagerly searching for clues while most other scientists kept far away from this area because so little was known about it, and the NIH was not at that time funding research grants devoted to lymphatics.

Assembling the equipment, reagents, staff, and timeline of experiments, I wrote copious plans on what experiments to conduct, thought about what theories I might offer with the potential results, designed statistical methods that would most appropriately analyze the data, planned a critical match of the data, and imagined how my experiments would be discussed with my colleagues and, somewhere in the future, how I would present the data at local, national, and international meetings and publish papers in peer-reviewed scientific journals.

What motivates one's excitement and fascination to scientific discovery? How do scientists make discoveries and so enhance human understanding? Most people would answer these questions by a simple answer: by observation and experiment. But observation is not a passive absorption of sensory information. What a scientist sees is usually a tiny part of what really exists, and it is not immediately possible to tell up front which observations are relevant and which are not. Experiment is not only seeing what happens when you change a few things around because they happen to be in the lab. To make accurate conclusions, one needs a third component, inference, or an aspect of the mind that can imagine connections amongst what is already known beyond doubt about a subject, hypothesize the next part of this topic or subject, and design experiments to confirm the "truth."

I had always wondered how people would react to my persistent questioning mind, and I had already experienced the reactions of my parents and neighbors to creating my first photographic enlargement in my darkroom, my medical school colleagues' reaction to my sickle cell thalassemia study, the surprise of my colleagues at UCLA when I discovered a new way to study monocytes in the peripheral blood of cancer patients, and the interest in a possible immune-suppressing protein in the blood of patients dying of many diseases including cancer. My motivations had often been misinterpreted, and I knew what it felt like to have journal editors reject papers, and all the uncertainty had made me wonder where in the range of the world of achievements or oblivion I would end up. I did not initially think about direct clinical applications for my anticipated studies, but I did anticipate that I would attract new students and establish my new home at Henry Ford Health System in a new light.

Pursuit of a scientific career was clearly not just a "job," and most surgeons spent their time in the operating room, having done a little research during their surgical internship and residency training, often for the sole reason of impressing their program directors sufficiently enough to get outstanding letters of recommendation, necessary to garner more interest from prestigious fellowship programs that offered more advanced surgical training. I had already spent much more time doing basic research than most other surgeons so that I could call myself a "physician-scientist."

Physician-scientists are often dedicated to exploring new medical knowledge and techniques by doing research work on various diseases, teaching students, and doing administrative and patient care in government or private institutions. The academic faculties in Pretoria, Johannesburg, Edinburgh, London, Chicago, Los Angeles, and Sacramento, where I had trained, differed from their private practice colleagues who devoted their time entirely to treating patients, running their practices, being involved in local politics, and avoiding big, time-consuming research efforts. The practice of a physician-scientist requires many skills besides clinical knowledge, including self-motivation, a dedication to work in challenging research situations, and an ability to manage multiple projects simultaneously. I realized I would need to have a high tolerance for failure and frustration while doing research work.

As a new investigator with limited local, national, or international recognition by peers, I was motivated to not only help patients and society, I quickly became aware of the weeding out process of research scientists, a process known to students of Darwinian natural selection. If my ideas weren't competitive enough to lure funding, my career as a scientist would end. I had no qualms about the competitive atmosphere amongst scientists in seeking prestige and personal reward, knowing that the poetic satisfaction of crucial institutional research support depended on hard work and ideas, and I was certainly up to the task. Besides, if I failed at research, I could always fall back on my surgical skills and earn a living somewhere operating on people.

The 1,800-square-foot research lab at Henry Ford Hospital had space for bench top and animal experiments and an office for me. I installed cell culture and cell freezing capabilities. The Fund for Henry Ford Hospital, initiated by Henry Ford II at the request of hospital administrators and funded by philanthropist and investor friends of Henry Ford, gave me enough money to continue to work for two years after which I would be expected to have my own funding from the National Institutes of Health or other outside sources. This process, like the tenure advancement systems of most research universities in North America, also gave me the security of a large patient population, and two lab techs, Patricia Westrick and Bernie Fox, who had worked with the previous director of Surgery Research. Later, I hired Lisa Nelson and Patricia Anaya, and we worked together like a well-oiled machine. At various times I hired undergraduate students from local universities for short summer stints. Many surgical residents, looking for a way to enhance their resumes, worked with me for short periods of time.

My life as a surgical scientist pulled me in a tug of war between my time in the lab, where I was in a building filled with full-time researchers, one of only a few physician-scientists doing laboratory research, and the nine-hundred-bed hospital and clinics filled with physicians dedicated to patient care and teaching where "research" meant clinical questions answered by observing and analyzing clinical conditions in patients and writing papers for clinical journals and publications designed for clinicians. To the surprise of many of my friends not familiar with the Henry Ford Health System, our Institute had almost as much funding in research as some of the medium-sized state universities.

The first objective of any surgical scientist is to think of an unresolved surgical problem, do library research to find out what other scientists are doing to solve the problem, and think of an idea to create a pathway of experiments to change the way the problem is managed. Having seen patients like Howard and Helen and many others who had all their lymph nodes removed when those nodes had no melanoma in them, and where common sense suggested they did not benefit from the operation, and as happened in a number of patients, they developed lymphedema, a severe lifelong complication that was incurable, a doctor-induced disease, I kept wondering if there was a way to determine which patients with melanoma had lymph-node metastasis when I first saw them. One of the first aspects of cancer management a medical student learns when examining a new cancer patient is to seek an answer to this question by examining the lymph nodes draining the cancerous organ.

Cancer that has spread to a regional lymph node causes that node to enlarge and feel hard. Melanoma that starts in the skin of the arm can metastasize to one or more of the lymph nodes in the ipsilateral armpit and become palpable to experienced fingers when they reach a large enough size. That size threshold varies depending on the weight of the patient, being easier to detect in thin patients where there is little interfering fat than in a morbidly obese patient. The enlarged and firm node is also easier to palpate when it is closer to the skin surface, while a deep node, even when quite big, is often missed by exploring fingers.

Even experienced physicians misinterpreted the existence of metastases in an armpit lymph node in about thirty percent of cases, and more sophisticated and sensitive methods were investigated to see whether surgical removal of all the nodes to find one involved could be avoided. Studies had already been done using CT, a computed tomography scan, a highly sophisticated radiologic imaging procedure that uses computer-processed combinations of many X-rays taken from different angles to produce cross-sectional images or virtual "slices" of scanned lymph nodes without cutting, allowing physicians to evaluate the size of those nodes. CT scans were more accurate at determining node size than the examining fingers of an experienced physician but not perfect enough to allow a definitive conclusion that the tumor had spread to the node. Besides, the detailed internal structure could not be deciphered by the CT scan, which could merely see whether the node was enlarged. If enlargement of a node always meant cancer, that might allow a more accurate use of the scan, but nodes were known to enlarge after infections, vaccinations, or for other non-malignant reasons. The conclusive diagnosis of metastasis was only made possible by removing all the nodes and subjecting them to painstakingly careful histologic evaluation by a trained pathologist. There was no way to identify and remove the first node to which a cancer would spread. Other radiologic tests and scans were neither sensitive nor specific enough to supplant surgical excision and pathologic review.

I realized quite early on that I needed an animal model of spontaneous lymph node metastasis to explore mechanisms by which cancers spread to lymph nodes. I reasoned that, by understanding more about how cancers metastasize to nodes, I might find a way in humans to remove only the one or two lymph nodes to which a melanoma had metastasized to the armpit, groin, or neck instead of removing all ten to fifty lymph nodes normally found in those lymph node stations.

I spent months reading published articles to find appropriate models. Since my first use of the Johannesburg library, and subsequent school and university libraries, I had developed a ritual where I spent many hours focusing my mind intensely on one subject, found a list of articles or textbooks on that topic, read them intensely while taking copious notes, drew lots of pictures and diagrams to help me remember the gist of the research and the concepts presented, and found other articles on related subjects by looking at the references and finding them. The process was much like a pilgrimage, a journey to an unknown or foreign place, with the purpose of searching for a new or expanded meaning of an area of interest; after which, the pilgrim returns enlightened to his daily life, sometimes enhancing the wisdom and understanding of others with his new ideas. I often found it difficult to keep focus on the topic because other topics lured me away, like the irresistible songs of the Sirens that lured inquisitive sailors to their death in Greek mythology.

My interest in finding an animal lymph node metastasizing model strengthened and began to keep my mind focused and, as days turned to weeks, and weeks turned to months, my mind became embedded in the quest for the elusive prototype. I looked at models of tumors in animals found spontaneously growing in domestic pets or in wild animals, which might be of interest to veterinarians but would not satisfy my needs. I needed a small rodent model, probably a mouse, in which I could rapidly grow the same tumor repeatedly and reliably, and that required a tumor that would grow in a genetically modified strain of mice whose immune systems would not reject the tumor. I also needed a tumor that could mimic the growth of a melanoma in Man, spreading to the nearest lymph node in the groin, armpit, or neck, and then to the lungs or other internal organs. Copious research in the library failed to help me find such a model.

The field of experimental metastasis had taken an interesting turn in the early 1970s when Fidler reported a model of melanoma that metastasized to the lung after intravenous injection of viable genetically identical melanoma cells into C57BL/6 mice. Scientists love quantitative experiments, and this model allowed the researcher to count the number of tumor nodules in mouse lungs after injecting a known number of tumor cells. I had read the papers and even heard Fidler speak at meetings, but it was only now, intensely interested in starting my own research, that I began to realize that I might develop a model myself. I argued with myself, since there was no one else in the institution to debate this issue, that Fidler's model, even though it had provided major new insights into metastasis, did not truly mimic the natural pathways of metastasis since tumors in animals, and Man did not normally enter blood vessels by injection through a needle but grew for a while in the tissues and spread to internal organs only after eluding the natural immunity at the primary site in the skin or other organs. It dawned on me that Fidler's mouse melanoma cells, which he called F10, might grow in the mouse foot pad and I hypothesized that they would metastasize to the lymph node behind the knee and, from there, in an orderly fashion, to the lymph node in the groin.

A "hypothesis" is an inspired guess, a creative act of mind, the product of a blaze of insight, a brainwave, and I do not quite understand how it arises. It comes as an imaginative preconception, and it comes from within to those who seek truth and want it to come, and to those whose minds are prepared and open to it. Most of the everyday business of biological sciences consists of testing experimentally the logical implications of hypotheses. To think ahead, to think of a research problem still to be solved comes naturally to most experienced scientists, and I can look back at how my ideas for the development of a spontaneously metastasizing mouse melanoma came to me while sitting in the library and thinking about how to create such a model was more a matter of luck or good fortune, without which I would surely have failed to produce a new idea.

In the world of the imagination, anything is possible.

Setting up experiments in mice at a time when the ethics of such experiments were seriously challenged by organizations who believed that nothing good came out of such experiments while destroying the lives of animals was my first hurdle and required approval of the Institutional Animal Care and Use Committee. In retrospect, the process of writing a proposal on the development of a mouse model was very good for me, but it did not feel like that then. Research committees require details, and one is forced to guess at those details when one doesn't know. I couldn't be sure the tumors would grow in mouse footpads let alone how long they would take to kill the animal. I didn't know for certain if the tumors would spread to the lymph nodes or how many would and how many would not. That was the experiment. The committee needed a justification of the number of mice needed, a perfectly reasonable request, but the formulas for assessing this information required information that no one had published, and I had to guess. How had Einstein predicted the sun's rays would be bent by gravity when nobody had reported that, and the proof came about fourteen years after his landmark paper in 1905?

Trying to do what no one had previously attempted is how scientists produce new ideas, but scientific progress and its translation to the fruits of technology are far from a linear process. We received the mouse melanoma cells from Fidler, but it took time for us to learn how to keep them alive in culture. We housed the mice in a well-organized animal care facility, but we soon discovered we could not use male mice because they terrorized each other in horrendous ways, reminiscent of what male felons do to each other in prisons, and we finally settled on female mice since they could live together in cages without fighting. We experimented with sedation medications, which were necessary for every interventional event, such as injecting tumor cells into the foot pad and measuring the diameter of the foot every Monday, Wednesday, and Friday. The veterinarian watched carefully over every step, and we had to sacrifice the mice rather than let them suffer when tumors grew to a certain size. Even the methods of sacrifice needed a little research, but we finally settled on a rapid, painless dose of carbon dioxide gas directly into sealed cages.

Phase two of our mouse experiments demanded that we find a way to remove the nodes behind the knee and in the groin, and the recognition that our hypothesis was correct; that the tumor did spread from the footpad to the lymph node behind the knee and, from there, to the femoral node in the groin, and, from there, to the lungs.

The emotional high one experiences the first time one sees one's hypothesis proven correct is an ethereal feeling, like the joyful triumph of Roger Federer's face and body when he hits the winning forehand drive at the Wimbledon tennis final. The first of a series of mouse autopsies clearly showed melanoma in the footpad and metastases in the popliteal lymph node behind and above the knee, but no metastases in the femoral lymph nodes or the lungs. After months of tweaking experimental variables, we discovered a consistent way to get lung metastases. We had produced a reproducible mouse model of melanoma metastasis. It was then that I felt triumphant for the first time.

Now we could investigate how metastases to lymph nodes occur.

Chapter 17

Unravelling Lymph Node Metastasis

How does one describe the feeling of triumph when a major experiment works and proves a hypothesis? Joy and wonder erupted in the lab when we discovered a way to reliably and repeatedly evaluate lymph node metastasis with the mouse model. As I recall the feelings that we had proved the model worked, and that my simple hypothesis had been correct, I think I was for weeks in a state of euphoria, a rare, exciting, oceanic, deeply moving, and exhilarating feeling of happiness, described by Maslow, the great American humanist psychologist as a "peak experience."

Scientific discovery seems to be a common trigger of the peak experience. Other triggers include art, nature, sporting triumphs, sex, creative work, and introspection. I felt blissful upon waking in the morning, eager to start another experiment, and my thoughts constantly reverberated around the relationship of the tumor in the footpad, the metastasis to the popliteal and femoral lymph nodes, and to the lungs. I dreamed about the model when sleeping at night and was fully immersed, completely absorbed, in the experiments we did, so much so that I sometimes lost a sense of time. According to Maslow the emotions of subjects feeling such peak experiences include worship, a sort of spiritual experience that one might feel when totally absorbed in communal religious practice, and I felt like there had to be some higher power that enlightened me.

At that time I was enthralled by Stanley Kubrick's thought-provoking 1968 movie *2001: A space Odyssey,* and although there was no uniform way to interpret the experiences of the sci-fi astronaut, Dave, and Earth's mission to Jupiter, I remembered the symbol of a granite obelisk appearing four times in the movie whenever a creative idea came to the characters' imagination. The first time the obelisk appears is when a primitive ape on the African landscape picks up a large bone from the skeleton of a dead animal and starts aimlessly playing with it, swinging it around until he accidentally hits one of the bones on the ground. He looks at the bone that he had just struck and then deliberately raises the bone he holds and strikes the other bone again, a little harder than he had done before. He repeats the action, hitting the target bone harder, and the next time, even harder, breaking the recipient bone. The granite obelisk appears next to him, suggesting a revelation has occurred, and "Thus spoke Zarathustra," the powerful music of Richard Strauss, fills the theater as the ape, suddenly realizing the significance of his action, demonstrates his immense ecstasy and roars excitedly, throwing his weaponized bone high in the air. In a later scene, having "armed" his fellow apes with large bones as weapons, he leads them in defeating a rival troupe of stronger apes that had not yet learned of the use of the weapons and thus wins back a watering hole that they had previously lost.

I felt that I had been enlightened by something like the Kubrick obelisk, giving me a new way to investigate how tumors spread to lymph nodes and to find out how those tumors traveled from the lymph nodes to the lungs. Ideas came rapidly, and I felt energized and alive, losing all sense of doubt and self-criticism, mindful of the present moment, free of inner conflicts, and functioning almost effortlessly every day at what seemed like an optimal level. Every new idea seemed perfect and doable. I think I sensed a new ability to perceive, accept, understand, and enjoy the journey of my life.

My first experiments with the new model looked at physical aspects of the process of lymph node metastasis. I had read reports of tumors in Minnesota frogs that spread to the lungs and killed the amphibian in summer when it was warm, but the tumor failed to metastasize in winter when it was cold. It was easy enough to suggest that high temperatures, hyperthermia, might make tumor cells metastasize more to lymph nodes and lungs, and we proved that to be true in the mouse model. But why?

The scientific mind is stirred by questions like this. Perhaps it is true of all of us, even those who claim that they're not scientists. There are so many "why" questions every day in our lives, from issues with the kitchen appliances to temporary disruption of television service to why the neighbor stopped watering his grass or why the gardener didn't show up at his usual time and many others. My questions were focused on observations in our new metastasis model, and since no-one else had ever used this model, every new observation could be followed and dissected. I began to explore the effects of heat on tumor cells growing in culture and to look at how heat in the intact mouse foot might affect the flow of lymph fluid towards the popliteal lymph node. I imagined that raising the temperature in the footpad would create larger volumes of fluid which, like a rapidly flowing river, would wash tumor cells more rapidly and in greater numbers towards the lymph nodes.

The lymph flow question prompted me to think about possible new technologies that would need collaboration with a physicist. At that time, nobody was seriously looking at the flow of lymph in animals, so I couldn't get on the telephone and call someone in another part of the country to get an easy answer.

Serendipity, the occurrence and development of events by chance in a happy or beneficial way, is so interesting a phenomenon when one thinks about moving forward to the next step not knowing how to accomplish that goal. I was unable to measure lymph flow myself, realizing that such measurement would be vitally important, I was wondering who to contact, perhaps a physicist who might be interested in the project, when suddenly, out of the blue yonder, within days of my idea, a young woman in need of a lab to do experiments for a PhD in medical physics at Oakland University appeared unannounced in my office. Mary Avery had started her course work towards a graduate degree in medical physics after getting a bachelor's degree in physics at Wayne State University. My friend, Fred Hetzel, a physicist in the radiation oncology department at Henry Ford Hospital, who taught part time at Oakland University, suggested to Mary that she talk to me about a project. She needed something unique and asked if I could help her. Since the lymph flow measurement was fresh on my mind, I suggested she work on a project to accurately measure lymph flow in mouse limbs, and she immediately jumped at the offer.

Months of physics formulas, ideas, and discussions followed, both Mary and I learning from each other, me learning more physics than I ever cared to know, she learning afresh about the physiology of the blood circulation that I knew as it related to clinical diseases and my extensive study of physiology in medical school. The result, like two sets of engineers building a tunnel from one side of a mountain to the other, from opposite ends, carefully planning to meet accurately in the middle, was a miraculous meeting of the minds, an overlap of expertise, like a Venn diagram, that resulted in a synergism that eventually led me and my UCLA mentor, Don Morton, to devise a new operation.

The decision to use methylene blue to outline otherwise invisible lymphatic trunks in the mouse leg was quite simple when Mary combined her physics knowledge with my clinical knowledge. She wanted to work out compartments in the mouse leg, and she needed to see the lymphatics. She suggested using a dye that would be absorbed into the lymphatic capillaries in the foot, and I suggested methylene blue because I knew the particle sizes needed for lymphatic absorption, and the blue dye fitted that well.

Terry Sarantou, a surgical resident working with me for a few months in the lab, also needed a project, and after Mary injected the blue dye and saw the lymphatics, I suggested he measure the diameters of lymphatic trunks in mice with and without tumors, hypothesizing that increased flow produced increased metastasis to the lymph nodes, as shown following heat treatment, and we also had discovered an association between the size of tumors in the footpad and the likelihood of spread to the node. Perhaps, I argued, the diameters of lymphatics are related to the size of the footpad tumors. And that is what we found. Another beautifully intuitive experiment that worked perfectly and led to never before noted associations and more sophisticated experiments, another opportunity for me to "float on a cloud," to feel a genuine triumph, a surge of productivity, and allowed Terry to enhance his resume and eventually head to Southern California to train with Morton. We also did further experiments showing that heating tumors in mice increased the diameters of lymphatic trunks while also increasing the lymph flow.

The "high" I felt continued. Think of the most wonderful experiences of one's life, the happiest, most ecstatic moments, moments of rapture, like being in love or a special feeling while listening to a musical piece that changes the brain or being suddenly mesmerized by a magnificent painting. That's how I felt every day for days, weeks, and months.

Mary needed a radioactive protein to accurately measure the rates of flow of lymph from the mouse footpad to the popliteal lymph node, and we settled on using technetium, already used in human patients to determine the direction of lymphatic drainage in melanoma patients. We injected the radiocolloid into the footpad and removed the popliteal lymph node at various timed periods and compared that in a sensing device, a gamma camera, attached to a computer, using algorithms set up by Mary and other physicists in the radiation oncology department, and observed and recorded the speed with which lymph flowed in the mouse lymphatic trunks. Later, using similar concepts in human patients, we calculated the rate at which lymph flowed in humans, finding that mice and Men did not differ much.

In the 1980s, the growing field of experimental metastasis, led by Fidler, focused heavily on biological changes in tumor cells that made them metastasize. Scientists reported many changes in the molecules and structures of malignant cells as they moved from growing in the anatomical place where they began, to invasion into the tissues and blood vessels to metastasis to internal organs in the host. No one paid much attention to mechanical factors involved in the process of spread. Cells moving in vitro along a chemically induced cascade, known as chemotaxis, and squeezing through tiny holes in pursuit of a chemo-attractant substance, certainly was seen and reported. But what about pressure inside the tumor, potentially "squeezing" tumor cells from one part to another? Instead of concentrating on cells being "pulled" towards a gradient of a chemo-attractant, I was interested in the "pushing" side. Since there was precious little intellectual energy directed at mechanical aspects of metastasis, I decided to investigate the physical components of tumor growth and spread.

After reading, reflecting, and discussing radiobiology with Fred, thinking about the patterns of growth of tumors exposed to radiation, and consulting Mary regarding the physics, we set up an elaborate series of experiments looking at the effects of different radiation doses on melanoma footpad growth, metastasis to lymph nodes and lungs, and the rates of lymph flow related to each of those parameters. Low doses of radiation, while slightly decreasing the growth of footpad tumors, increased lymph flow, and metastasis, while higher radiation doses markedly decreased footpad tumor growth, lymph flow, and metastases.

In the meantime, I also had a clinical practice where I operated on melanoma patients, deciding on whether to remove all the lymph nodes, complete radical lymphadenectomy, based upon what the tumor looked like under the microscope. I imagined there was a genetic predisposition to lymph node metastasis, but no one had yet identified such genes. Instead, we relied on the pathologist by examining the way the tumor cells oriented themselves in the tissues to tell us how likely it was that the melanoma would spread to the lymph nodes. Patients undergoing complete radical lymphadenectomy whose lymph nodes did not contain melanoma metastasis were very happy, but some of them developed chronic lymphedema, reinforcing my need to find a way to identify which lymph node was the first to receive lymph from the primary tumor in the skin.

It wasn't only the skin tumors that bothered me. My breast cancer practice also increased during that time, and some of my patients in that group developed chronic lymphedema after lymphadenectomy. I could take my clinical experience and questions to the lab, what became known as "bed to benchtop," and bring lab experimental findings back to patients, known as "back to the bedside." That prompted me to realize that some of my lab questions could be better addressed in patients in the operating room. So it was that I discovered the work of Rakesh Jain, Director of the E.L. Steele Laboratories for Tumor Biology at the Massachusetts General Hospital.

Professor Jain, a chemical engineer by training, ran a course on tumor physiology in Boston that revolutionized my thinking about the mechanics of metastasis. I took a simple technique for measuring interstitial fluid pressure in tumors from Jain's teaching course and set up a system in the operating room on the fourth floor of the Henry Ford Hospital and observed and recorded pressures in human breast cancer, benign conditions of the breast and normal breast tissues, and found that the pressure inside cancers was much higher than normal, confirming what Jain had already discovered in other tumors in animals. This intriguing finding set me to asking "why" again.

A good hypothesis looks for an explanation of whatever needs to be explained and the art of devising a hypothesis can be tested by practical experiments. Most of the daily business of scientists consists of testing experimentally the logical implications of the hypothesis. Jain and his mentor, Gullino at the National Cancer Institute, had extensively studied the formation of interstitial fluid in rodent tumors and pathologists at the Harvard Medical School found a protein in tumors that caused fluid in blood coursing through a tumor to leak out of the vessels into the surrounding tissues, resulting in a higher volume of fluid and resultant increase in pressure.

We had measured lymphatic flow from mouse tumors and found it to be higher than from normal tissues, and that seemed to fit with the finding of increased pressure in tumors. My mind thinks visually and simply, and I imagined the tumor was like a pump that caused fluid to travel more quickly to the regional lymph nodes. Everything I was studying, in the lab and in the clinic, seemed to corroborate my ideas about mechanical causes of metastasis but this worried me. As a seeker of truth, I was concerned that I might have become so sure of my mechanical hypothesis that I would be unable to see other truths. I had lots of experience in the lab and in the clinic, but I had not received formal instruction in scientific methods that graduate doctoral students have. I indulged in imaginative guesswork and had already recognized another truth about the scientific process: those with doctoral graduate degrees in science did not seem to do better than physicians.

Scientists are often reluctant to shake off received beliefs and sometimes feel impatient of ideas that fall outside a prevailing paradigm, and my research was not a popular way of looking at the problem of metastasis. I worried that my ideas would dry up if I didn't push them hard. But my mentor and friend Don Morton changed my direction in the lab and encouraged me to focus on a practical side of my discoveries.

Chapter 18

The Sentinel Node in Melanoma

Morton, always friendly to his trainees, visited my poster at the annual meeting of the Society of Surgical Oncology in 1989 in Atlanta. He seemed unusually interested in my mouse melanoma project, asking me questions about the methylene blue injection to outline the lymphatic trunks and the studies I had done using radioactive technetium to study rates of lymphatic flow in mice and in patients. Two years later, he published an article on blue dye injection in cats to find the lymph node in the groin, and he invited me to lunch at the SSO meeting in Chicago.

"The sentinel node is big, David, and it will become even bigger," he said.

"The sentinel node?"

"It's a word used to describe a lymph node that acts as the entry site of tumor cells into the lymph nodes in the neck, axilla, or groin. It's like the word 'sentry' in the Civil War prisoner-of-war camps," he said. "We injected blue dye into the skin of 223 melanoma patients and found the node in 194 cases who were undergoing lymphadenectomy, and thirty-four patients had metastases. It is time for us to do a prospective study in patients, and I'm hoping you will join me and eight other centers around the world in a study."

"What do I need to do?" I asked.

"We'll submit a program project grant to the National Cancer Institute, and I'll need your resume," he said. "I'll mail you the proposal. Each center will have a principal investigator, and you will need to get Internal Review Board approval. To make sure that each investigator at every center is able to find the correct sentinel node, we will do thirty cases each to start and a committee will review the success rate of each surgeon. If you manage to find the sentinel node in greater than 95 percent of cases, you'll go onto the randomized part of the study."

So started the Multicenter Selective Lymphadenectomy Trial, or MSLT. It was designed to determine whether removal of one or two lymph nodes in select cases with melanoma could replace removing all the nodes in that lymph node basin in the neck or the armpit or the groin. It was the idea that had popped into my mind when I had trained in Los Angeles with Morton and I saw patients develop lymphedema after lymphadenectomy. It was the idea that motivated the development of the mouse melanoma model. Morton had taken it one step further, a step that I had not taken yet but which I was headed towards in my mind, the obvious step if one wanted to avoid lymphedema in patients.

I had mixed feelings when I thought about this important study. On the one hand, I wanted to be the pioneer in this effort, and I had an initial selfish feeling that I had been beaten to the finishing gate by my revered teacher. But scientific collaboration is not at all like cooks elbowing each other from the pot of broth. Nor is it like artists working on the same canvas. Although having an idea can be very personal, it is also evident from the history of science that it is the atmosphere that one member of the team sparks off the others and helps them develop and build on each other's ideas. In this case, what mattered was that something important had been thought of and that Morton must have known that I had thought of the idea as well, or he would not have invited me to be part of this international effort.

Collaboration connotes a joint effort, and like synergism, it suggests that the joint effort is greater than the sum of the several contributions to it. Collaboration is a joy when it works, and it only works well when there is some generosity of spirit. I would have contractual obligations to Morton and the team, and I could at least continue my lab research looking into the mechanisms of lymph node metastasis and information from the study might enhance my own studies.

The challenge of an NCI-funded program project for me was the bureaucracy, not the science. As a surgeon, one is scrutinized daily by the operating room staff, the patient's family, and the surgical residents and medical students in training. If one does something wrong, it is soon discovered by the way the patient recovers from the operation. Being an investigator in an international study adds immensely to the paperwork and the potential for audits by visiting inspectors. Unlike a major research university where there are layers of data collectors and administrators, research nurses, and other personnel, and where the surgeon in a study like the MSLT is assisted in his or her efforts, the set-up at Henry Ford Health System was relatively thin and understaffed. I had nobody to help me prepare for and manage all the extra work required.

Fortunately, I had "slush" funds from a grateful patient, a wealthy lawyer from Grand Rapids whose threatening thigh tumor I had successfully treated, and I was able to hire Lynne Wachna, a nurse with the same kinds of obsessive instincts to excellence as I, to help manage the study with me.

The excitement and fascination of doing a new surgical procedure that has not been done in one's city or in the state where one lives is hard to describe but must feel something like climbing a mountain and not knowing what one will find at the top because no one has been there before. First, I had to get permission from the chief of General Surgery and the chairman of the surgery department, both of whom were highly skeptical of the procedure at the start. They thought it was fine to do a few cases, if it didn't cost the department any money and urged me to make sure I had the right approvals and consent forms so that I wouldn't create a legal nightmare for the department. Most surgeons who do research have trained personnel to review the consent for an experimental procedure, and I undertook the lengthy extra process, going through each sentence of the eight-page form with every patient.

The "M" in MSLT could also have meant "multidisciplinary," because the coordination on the day of surgery required a visit to the nuclear medicine department early in the morning, injection of the same radio-colloid we had used in mice, a gamma camera picture revealing the approximate site of the sentinel lymph node, a radiologist marking the spot on the skin, and a transfer to the operating room where the procedure was to be done.

My heart beating fast, I injected methylene blue around the melanoma site as I sought to find my first sentinel node in a human patient. No one had more experience finding the sentinel node in mice, but that didn't help me with the patient. Using the mark made by the radiologist on the patient's skin and a gamma probe that senses the radioactivity emanating from the sentinel node, I made an incision more carefully than usual and opened the tissues, going deeper and deeper, looking for a blue lymphatic that would lead me to the node. I think I stopped breathing, concerned that I would cut the delicate lymphatic, causing the dye to leak out and ruin my chances of finding the true sentinel node. In that state of mind, everything seemed to stand still, and every noise and movement appeared to be blotted out. I imagined what it must have been like for great inventors when they first tried out their inventions. What did Alexander Graham Bell feel when he spoke to his assistant the first time on the telephone? How did the lookout on Christopher Columbus's ship feel when he first saw land after crossing the Atlantic Ocean?

I needn't have worried because there it was! A stark contrast to the surrounding tissues, the tiny blue lymphatic led me down to a blue-stained lymph node, which registered the radioactivity from the radiologist-injected radio-colloid.

"Hot and blue," I yelled.

Smiles are hidden behind surgical masks, but the triumph registers in the eyes and the body language. Everything had worked according to plan and the sentinel node was removed and sent to the pathologist who also had a new procedure to undertake on the node, according to the protocol demanded for the study. Instead of the usual one or two slides to sample the node after removal, which had sufficed for the usual lymphadenectomy yielding ten to fifty nodes, the pathologist had agreed to do ten slides on one node, cutting the node in this agreed way as part of the study. Also new and different.

The MSLT study catapulted me into a new level of collaboration and involvement, preparing me clinically for a new era in melanoma management, eventually achieving the logical outcome that I had dreamed of for decades. Only a small number of patients with melanoma needed to have all their lymph nodes removed, saving many people from the dreadful complication of lymphedema. If only Helen and Howard had their melanomas thirty years later than they did.

Chapter 19

Paraguay and the Sentinel Node

Penile cancer is uncommon, but when it is diagnosed, it is psychologically devastating to the patient and often presents a challenge to the urologist. In rural Paraguayan farm workers, the surgical treatment for this disease, which included removing all the lymph nodes in both groins, caused unmanageable lifelong swelling, lymphedema, of both legs. The major problem in treating these patients was that lymphedema predisposed them to repeated life-threatening infections in the skin and soft tissues, cellulitis, of the legs, which in most cases barred them from returning to work on the farms where the risk of cellulitis while working in mud and with farm machinery was much higher than in cleaner jobs in cities. The farm workers who cannot work in the fields are economically ostracized, and they and the families they support may be doomed to lifelong poverty.

From 1968 through 1977, Cabanas, a little-known urologist, partially trained in the United States, did some astonishing studies in a rural part of Paraguay, his home country, to help farm workers with penile cancer avoid lymphedema so they could return to work after surgery without fear of recurrent infections. The way he set about doing these amazing studies led him to describe the sentinel node. I hadn't heard about his studies when we started our mouse studies in the 1980s because I didn't read the urology literature, or articles in Spanish, and finding such name associations, easily done many years later after the introduction of search engines like Google, required more directed library research than anyone did in this discipline at that time.

Cabanas's studies were even more astonishing because they were done using relatively unsophisticated technology, relying on simple X-rays coupled with injection of a radio-opaque dye into lymphatics in the penis, or lymphangiography. I tried to imagine what it must be like to volunteer to have a doctor inject a blue dye into the penis, waiting fifteen minutes until bluish lines appear on the top of the penis, and inserting a plastic cannula into the dye-filled lymphatics after cutting through the skin, followed by injection of a substance opaque to X-rays. Perhaps a man with cancer of the penis could be persuaded to have this done, in the hope that the doctor knew what he was doing and that this would somehow help heal him. But normal volunteers without any disease of the penis? Maybe Cabanas had a persuasive way that others might not have had. He would not have been able to do this kind of study in the United States, particularly in modern times where he would have needed a lengthy consent form and approval of a hospital Internal Review Board.

Having served on the Henry Ford Health System IRB for several years, I tried to imagine the dismay of the committee members if they were asked to review Cabanas's proposal. The chairman of the committee would have distributed proposals to individual members, and as "primary reviewer," I would have read the proposal, written an extensive review, and summarized my findings to the committee, pointing to the importance of the scientific question, the likelihood that the study could be completed as presented, the source of funding, the adequacy of the proposed statistical analysis, the human rights aspects, and the long-term social, cultural, and intellectual advances that might occur.

At that time, Joseph Shore was director of research and a recipient of many NIH grants. I imagined how he would question me if we had reviewed Cabanas's proposal.

"Did I understand that he planned to recruit normal men, without any disease of the penis, to subject themselves to a procedure where a physician would inject a blue dye into their penis and make a cut in the skin close to that injection site, insert a plastic cannula into a lymphatic, followed by injection of a dye, and have X-rays taken of the pelvis to show the position of a lymph node in relation to the bones of the pelvis?" asked Shore.

"Yes, that's the process."

"And these are normal men with no disease of the penis?"

"Yes."

"Does it hurt?"

"I presume it does."

"How long does it take the wound on the penis to heal?"

"Probably a week to ten days."

"During which time the patient is unable to have sex?"

"Probably not."

"How about passing urine?"

"That would probably not be a problem."

"Is there a chance of complications from the procedure?"

"I'm pretty sure that any cut anywhere in the body can result in excess bleeding and a potential for infection."

"What's the worst thing that can happen to the volunteer?"

"Well, Cabanas doesn't mention this, but I suppose he could get an infection with a bug that causes gangrene, which could theoretically result in amputation."

"How does Cabanas find normal volunteers for this study?"

"He doesn't say."

"Does he pay them?"

"He doesn't say."

"What if he doesn't find any volunteers?"

"He can't do the study."

"Let's say he does manage to find men to volunteer, how will this help patients with cancer of the penis?"

"He would do lymphangiography in the patient the same way he learned to do it on volunteers, and he would identify a lymph node in the groin by taking an X-ray in the operating room and removing that node, which he calls 'the sentinel node.'"

"What is the significance of the sentinel node?"

"After removing that node from both the left and right side of the groin, he would ask a pathologist to determine whether the tumor had spread there."

"How often does that tumor spread to the sentinel node?"

"Cabanas believes about 30 percent of the time."

"Okay. So, let's say the node has tumor in it. What then?"

"He would remove all the other lymph nodes from the groin and the lower pelvis."

"How does that differ from the standard way to treat cancer of the penis now?"

"The standard way now is to remove all the lymph nodes from both sides. If he only removes these nodes from the 30 percent with metastases in the sentinel lymph node, the remaining 70 percent would not have their nodes removed."

"What is the advantage of not having the rest of the nodes removed?"

"Only patients who have all the nodes removed are at risk of getting chronic swelling of the legs."

"How bad is chronic swelling of both legs?"

"It can be bad. The patients have to wear compression stockings for the rest of their lives, and they are at risk of getting cellulitis from the slightest injury."

"Cellulitis?"

"Yes, that's an infection which spreads quickly and may kill the patient if they don't get the appropriate antibiotics in time. Cabanas wants to save seven of every ten farm workers from getting this problem."

"You think we should approve this study?"

"It's a neat idea and, if it works, it could be useful in other cancers."

"Other cancers?"

"Yes. Lymphedema is a problem in patients with breast cancer and melanoma, and they are much more common than penile cancer. I think Cabanas's idea is unique and could produce a new paradigm of thinking."

I imagine many IRB members would have objected to this study because it seemed crude, and it may have been rejected after voting by the committee. But Cabanas reported his results in 1977 and showed the concept of an anatomically constant "sentinel node" to be solid; the lymph node with metastasis was often the only node involved, and patients who avoided radical removal of their remaining nodes remained free of recurrences.

By the time I discovered Cabanas and his study, we were already well into trying to prove the same concept in breast cancer.

Chapter 20

On the Shoulders of Giants

New ideas in science and medicine, like other changes that occur in how we all conceive of the world through change, become accepted through a complex process of social and intellectual consolidation. We see more and further than our predecessors, not because we have keener vision, better brains, or greater height but because we are privileged to have mentors, teachers, and thought leaders who have gone before us provide insights and ideas to be lifted up on their gigantic stature. In this way, each new generation discovers truths by building on previous discoveries.

By standing on the shoulders of giants we can see further, as articulated by Isaac Newton in the seventeenth century. Intellectual progress is gained by studying the works of major thinkers who have gone before us. Scholars in the thirteenth century paid tribute to Greek and Roman scholars. Thomas Aquinas, an immensely influential Catholic priest and theologian who considerably influenced Western thought, embraced several ideas put forward by Aristotle sixteen hundred years before him and attempted to synthesize Aristotelian philosophy with the principles of Christianity. This "scholasticism" so influenced society that students could not enter the great universities in France, England, or other countries without first mastering Aristotle.

I could easily acknowledge the work of Cabanas in identifying the sentinel node concept, and Gould, a surgeon from Washington, DC, who predated Cabanas by a decade and may have invented the term "sentinel node" in the management of parotid gland tumors. However, all of us working as pioneers in this field in the 1980s and 1990s had not even heard of Cabanas or Gould when we thought of the same idea independently. It may have resulted from a general tendency for all of us to be influenced by many things in the universe which affect our thinking all the time, perhaps even at the same time. Someone once said: "If a butterfly sneezes in Brazil, someone may catch a cold in Minnesota," perhaps a little simplistic and hard to imagine, but it does speak to similar ideas or events that seem to originate independently at the same time and may be related. My own interest in lymph nodes was heavily influenced by Morton while I trained with him at UCLA, but I was primed by my prior experiences and interest in the lymphatic system starting in childhood. Morton translated what we all knew in the 1990s into a practical way of performing sentinel node biopsy in melanoma at a time when I was heavily invested in finding how tumor cells metastasized to those nodes. I didn't have the wisdom or insight to translate what Morton translated because I was so interested in discovering why tumors spread to lymph nodes in the first place.

The giants whose shoulders I stood upon were not only Morton, Cabanas, and Gould but also other teachers and mentors in my training and in my reading. Without my real face-to-face teachers, like Tobias, Myburgh, Duplessis, Fahey, Morton, and Jain, and my patients with lymphedema, I might have devoted my time to other pursuits. There were also those whose works I studied and whose ideas I developed, and one of the most influential when I looked for reasons why tumor cells metastasize was Stephen Paget.

The son of James Paget, one of the founders of modern pathology in Victorian England and the nephew of a prominent Cambridge professor of medicine, and probably influenced by both, Stephen studied the case files of 735 women who had died of breast cancer. Until then, physicians believed that cancer spreads like an ink stain, spreading outward from a central mass of malignant tissue, a widespread belief that prompted William Halsted in Baltimore to initiate the use of radical mastectomy to treat breast cancer, an operation that stimulated surgeons everywhere to perform this operation and other radical operations on various organs starting in the 1890s extending through the first three-quarters of the twentieth century. To Paget, metastases did not appear to spread like an ink stain but rather to anatomically distinct distant sites, in non-random fashion, with a preference for some organs, such as the liver, lungs, bone, and brain. He was intrigued by places that seemed inhospitable to metastases, like the spleen, and certain bones, like those in the hands and feet. He coined the term "seed and soil," the cancer cell being the seed, the local environment within an organ being the soil. What intrigued me as well was that some people seemed to have organs, a "soil," more hospitable to metastases than in other people with the same tumor. Paget sowed a seed in my brain, except that I already had another seed growing there: the lymph system and the lymph nodes. I came to focus my passions on lymph node metastasis in breast cancer.

The Multidisciplinary Breast Cancer Tumor Board and clinic that I initiated in 1992 had started to flourish about the same time as the American College of Surgeons Oncology Group in Chicago, a National Cancer Institute-funded organization, started funding surgeons doing group cancer studies, and my colleague Armando Giuliano at the John Wayne Cancer Center introduced a major national study of sentinel node biopsy in breast cancer. This, for me, was another example of a fortunate, perhaps serendipitous, concatenation of events since I had separate funding from the NCI to study mechanisms of lymph node metastasis in my mouse model. My mind was filled with lymph nodes. I handled lymph nodes in the day, from both mice and patients, and dreamed about lymph nodes at night.

Like I had done for the MSLT in melanoma, I had to first prove to the researchers in Chicago that I was able to find the sentinel node in the armpits of selected breast cancer patients and make sure that my surgical colleagues at HFHS could also do the procedure accurately.

In every profession and in every walk of life there are examples of adventurers and explorers, and people who indulge in adventures and exploration are often thought of as courageous, doing something new, going to places where no one has been before. In modern history, we know of geographic firsts, such as reaching the South and North Poles, or the top of Mount Everest, technical feats such as the first man-made flights of the Wright brothers, the construction of the first steam engines, cotton gins, automobiles, space flights, reaching the moon, the broadcasting of radio conversations, television, the movies, and many more. In medicine, in the twentieth century, blood transfusion, antibiotics, vaccinations, heart-lung machines, electrocardiograms, X-rays, DNA, chemotherapy, joint replacements, organ transplantation, and many others had already changed the face of healing and disease management.

Sentinel node biopsy, although it initially didn't seem as life changing as all the other major advances in medicine, even after I discovered Cabanas's method of using sentinel node biopsy, slowly began to emerge as a major advance in the surgical treatment of melanoma in the 1990s. Some surgeons began to talk about using the procedure to manage breast cancer. Nobody knew how to do sentinel node biopsy in breast cancer, but we all thought that we should start by using the same blue dye and radiocolloid injections into the breast as we had used in melanoma. Since we didn't know exactly where in the breast to inject these tracing agents, we thought that we should inject adjacent to the cancerous tumor in the breast. The only problem was that we couldn't see or feel the tumor in some cases, and the precise site of injection required finding the tumor with imaging devices, like ultrasound, not easily done by surgeons untrained in that technology. That was when serendipity, or luck, visited again.

My first human sentinel node biopsy in a breast cancer patient in 1994, the first at Henry Ford Hospital, the first in the State of Michigan, differed from those I had done for melanoma because the blue dye injection deep in the lower outer quadrant of the breast was immediately followed by me seeing a blue lymphatic visible through the skin and heading towards the nipple area. The invisible lymphatic was made visible by the blue dye. Within a few minutes, the dye, again visible through the skin in a lymphatic trunk in the upper outer quadrant of the breast, started flowing towards the armpit at about the ten o'clock position of the right breast. My mind connected with my anatomy teaching days in Johannesburg where I had stumbled across the beautiful detailed drawings of the lymph channels in the breast by Sappey, and I remembered how he had clearly shown a major lymphatic trunk in the same area heading towards the lymph nodes in the axilla.

That observation got me thinking about how the breast might differ from the skin in all other parts of the body. The procedure of sentinel node biopsy in melanoma, a tumor of the skin, had shown us that it mattered immensely where the blue dye was injected. If we injected even an inch away from the melanoma, the dye would go to the wrong lymph node and not the true sentinel node. That inaccuracy would give the wrong information to the doctor and the patient. Accurate injection and tracing in melanoma became known as "lymphatic mapping," analogous to using a map to find the correct address. The breast seemed different, and I did an experiment to prove this in about one hundred patients with breast cancer as we moved more and more into doing the ACOSOG Z0010 study with Giuliano. My study helped me prove that it did not matter where in the breast I injected the tracing dyes; they ended up in the same lymph node in the armpit. A dye injected in the middle of the breast ended up in Sappey's plexus under the areola and then into the major lymphatic trunk at ten o'clock on the right side and two o'clock on the left side. It didn't seem to matter if the dye was injected into the skin or deep into the breast tissue, except when injected in the upper outer quadrant of the breast, where the dye would go directly into the lymphatic trunk and not into Sappey's subareola plexus.

Within fifteen years of the first efforts at doing the sentinel node biopsy, the surgery for breast cancer changed dramatically. In the 1980s, at least 60 percent of patients began to have only the lump of breast cancer removed without removing the whole breast, but they continued to have all the lymph nodes removed from the armpit. After it became apparent that breast cancer metastasized to the sentinel lymph node in about 25 percent of cases, only those patients with metastases had all the remaining lymph nodes removed, like Cabanas had described for the penis. A later series of studies showed that even those patients with sentinel lymph node metastases could sometimes safely avoid having the rest of the nodes removed.

While the art of portraiture has not been replaced by photography, and the chemically bleached, devitaminized or revitiminized, steam-baked, pre-sliced, mass-produced bread is not necessarily better than the old-fashioned crusty loaf of Grandma's bread, in science the present devours the past. I had found myself deeply absorbed in digesting the past, connecting the young me with the older me, filling my days with a sense of delight and watching the age of modern medicine evolve while the old-fashioned world of medicine disappeared.

I watch as the world of the sentinel node, because of many researchers, including me, has taken over the management of breast cancer and melanoma and is starting to do the same with other cancers. I remember patients treated with radical operations suffering long-term side effects, patients like Howard and Helen, and friends like Arlene, whose suffering might have been avoided if we had invented the sentinel node concept earlier, and I often wonder what will happen in the next twenty years when we could well see even this magnificent operation, the sentinel node biopsy, disappear, replaced by the new era of targeted and immune therapies.

What will not disappear is the excitement and fascination of scientific discovery, a process which enabled me to become a seeker after truth. That process is traceable to the repeatedly lucky exposure to mentors and teachers and learning from an early age to be present and aware of new ideas and their potential.

One can only advance knowledge by staying alert, curious, keeping an open mind and listening to those that were there before us.

Chapter 21

A Surgical Revolution Unfolds

Sally burst into tears when I entered the examination room sixteen years after I had done a complete axillary lymphadenectomy on the right side for breast cancer. This time, she had a new tumor in the left breast, and a needle biopsy showed invasive cancer.

"Hi, Sally," I said. "I'm so sorry that you have another cancer."

"I can't go through this again," she said.

"But I thought you did so well the last time. The surgery went well. The radiation to your breast seemed easy enough. You didn't need chemotherapy. The hormonal pill the medical oncologist gave you had no side effects. It should be easy enough for you to go through again, don't you think?"

"Do you see this arm, Doctor?" she asked.

She had moderate swelling of the right arm from the lymphadenectomy.

"I know you have lymphedema, but you seem to have it under control."

She took a deep breath, narrowed her eyes, tightened her facial muscles, wiped the tears from her cheeks, and looked at me directly.

"You don't have a clue how terrible this arm swelling is. It is always with me, morning, afternoon, and night." She took off the elastic stocking from her right arm and showed me the ridges of skin, the swollen fingers.

"Is it uncomfortable? Painful?" I asked.

"No pain. Just a slight pressure. I can't use my arm properly."

"What do you mean by properly?" I asked.

"It feels heavy all the time. When I want to take dishes out of the dishwasher, I'm always worried I'm going to drop them. The hand feels weaker than it used to be. The swelling seems to get in the way when I try to button my blouse. I must be careful what I do with my right hand. I can't wash the dishes in the sink without a thick protective glove. Forget about gardening. I used to love using my bare hands in my garden to pull weeds and to plant bulbs. I never worried about tiny cuts, abrasions, and insect bites. But one day I got a terrible infection in the right arm from an insect bite. It nearly killed me. I had to be in the hospital for days with intravenous antibiotics. Even simply dressing and undressing is a chore, every day."

"I think I understand your concern. You're worried because you think you need to have all your lymph nodes removed from your left armpit, and that you'll have lymphedema of the left arm. Well, I have good news for you."

I stopped briefly, giving her a moment to take in my last statement, and hoping that she would interrupt me and ask me what I was talking about.

She looked at me expectantly, waiting for me to continue.

"What if I told you that you probably don't need all your lymph nodes removed?"

"I don't understand. Last time you removed all the lymph nodes, and the tumor had not spread to any of them. And I got lymphedema. All these years I've wondered why you had to remove the lymph nodes if they didn't have tumor in them. Now you're telling me I didn't need to have them removed?"

"Things have changed a lot since your last surgery. We were just beginning to study a technique called sentinel lymph node biopsy, or SLNB. Studies have been done in North America, the United Kingdom, Europe, Asia, and Australasia on tens of thousands of women with breast cancer. We now know that it is safe to remove only one or two nodes from the armpit without removing the rest of them in most cases."

"Why didn't you do that on the right side?" she asked.

"We didn't know it was safe and effective at that time," I said. "And we didn't know how to do it. We had to work out a technique."

"I see. So how do I know that it is okay for me this time?"

"Because of the studies I mentioned. The technique is now the standard way to treat invasive cancer."

"Last time I think you took out more than twenty lymph nodes. Do I have the same number on the left side?"

"Yes, probably about the same number."

"How do you know which lymph node to take out and which to leave?"

"The day of your surgery you will get an injection of a radioactive solution into your breast. Then we take you into the operating room, give you a general anesthetic, inject a blue dye into your breast, and make a cut across the armpit. I look for a blue lymphatic and follow it to a blue lymph node deep in the axilla. We have a small gamma probe, about the size of a small cucumber, that measures the radioactivity in the same lymph node. We know this is the correct node if it is hot from the radioactivity and blue from the blue dye, and we take it out, send it to the pathologist, and sew up your incision."

"What happens after the surgery? Last time there was no pain in the breast from removing the cancerous lump, but the pain in the armpit was terrible. I had to take oxycodone for days, and I hate that stuff. And I couldn't raise my arm above my shoulders for months. And I was numb under the arm for years. And then I got lymphedema."

"Yes, I remember. Most patients these days who have the SLNB have no pain at all. I mean none. I give everyone a prescription for an analgesic, and 80 percent don't take even one pill, and those who do need something may take one or two pills for the pain. That's it."

"Does this new operation cause lymphedema?" she asked.

"I have not seen any patients with lymphedema after SLNB," I said, "but some surgeons have reported a small number of patients with mild swelling."

"How about the shoulder stiffness? That was bad, and I did physical therapy for months to help me get back to being able to raise my arm to get supplies out of the top shelf in my kitchen."

"No, not at all. No limitation of movement," I said.

"How about that numbness in the armpit?" she asked.

"The nerve that brings sensation from the armpit to the spinal cord, and the brain runs right through the middle of the cluster of axillary lymph nodes.

When we remove all the lymph nodes, we take that nerve. When we remove the sentinel lymph node, we try to avoid cutting or injuring the nerve. I have seen a few patients in whom there has been damage to the nerve, but it is nowhere near as obvious as when we do a complete lymphadenectomy."

By this time, Sally seemed much less anxious, and she was relieved to get surgical treatment that sounded to her like it would be much easier than her first operation.

"One last question, Doctor. You know I have grandchildren, and I want to be there to help my daughters and to be there for their kids. They need me to help with babysitting and other stuff. My other cancer didn't come back. How can I be sure that this operation to take out only one or two lymph nodes will be as good?"

"The data from multiple studies is convincing. Patients do just as well with the smaller operation as they used to do with the larger operation. That's why we do it with confidence. That is why it has become the standard operation for breast cancer."

"Do you think I should have both my breasts removed? I'm sick and tired of having mammograms every year."

"I haven't pushed you in that direction, but this is a question that I get from many patients in your position. Let's talk about this option a little so you can see where I'm coming from."

"Well, I'm worried about getting another cancer in my breasts."

"Yes, I know. This is a little concerning. The chances are relatively small, but you are at risk for recurrence. You would be at much higher risk if you had a genetic mutation. That would push me a little harder, and I might even have suggested a mastectomy up front. But we know you don't have a gene mutation. By the way, all the studies showing that SLNB is safe and effective were done in patients undergoing lumpectomy to treat the breast cancer. The studies did not include patients who have a mastectomy. If you have a mastectomy instead of a lumpectomy, we would take out the sentinel lymph node and have the pathologist look at it while you are under anesthetic. If the lymph node shows metastatic tumor, we would need to remove all the other axillary lymph nodes."

"Oh, no! Really?"

"Yes, I'm afraid so.'

"Okay, then let's plan to do a lumpectomy and take out the sentinel lymph node. Now, you're sure I don't have to have all the rest of my armpit lymph nodes removed even if the sentinel node is positive?"

"Yes, I'm pretty sure, except if there are a number of other nodes near the sentinel node that feel suspicious and we remove them and find that there is tumor in them too. But we would not do the complete lymphadenectomy until after we discuss the final pathology report with you when you return to the clinic after the surgery. In other words, we are not planning to have the pathologist look at the sentinel node while you're still under general anesthetic."

Sally had her lumpectomy, with the SLNB, and her lymph node was negative. She had radiation and did not need chemotherapy, and took a hormone manipulating drug for five years, and now, nine years later, she is doing well with no signs of breast cancer recurrence.

Meanwhile, studies in patients with melanoma had shown results like those in breast cancer. The results and conclusions of the MSLT studies initiated and managed by Morton saved many patients from having radical lymphadenectomies. Similar studies in the United Kingdom, Australia, Italy, France, Germany, and Switzerland showed that most patients with melanoma who had SLNB did not need to have all the lymph nodes from the draining cluster of nodes removed, even when the node had metastatic tumor.

Grace was a recent example of a melanoma patient with a lower limb melanoma who escaped the consequences of a complete groin lymphadenectomy. An elegant woman in her late fifties, she developed a melanoma in the nailbed of the left large toe and was referred to me not long ago. She would have needed all her groin lymph nodes removed in an era before the development of the sentinel node biopsy, and she was terrified that's what she would need because she had a friend I had operated upon for melanoma of the calf in the 1990s who had a complete groin lymphadenectomy and had developed such bad lymphedema that she couldn't wear her clothes as before, embarrassed to wear skirts or dresses because the thick elastic stocking she wore to treat the lymphedema was so unattractive.

I remembered her friend as soon as Grace started talking about her and told me she didn't want the same to happen to her. She wanted to be able to wear a suit to work with "normal" stockings. This was so important that she continued the conversation by asking me if I could just treat the toe and forget about removing the nodes in her groin.

"It's very important that we know whether the melanoma has spread to the lymph nodes in the groin," I said.

"Why?" asked Grace.

"We don't need to remove all the lymph nodes anymore. We just need to remove the sentinel lymph node."

"Yes, I read something about the sentinel node. I Googled it when I heard there had been a change in the treatment of melanoma. Is it true that only one out of every five patients with melanoma have metastases in the node?"

"Yes, that is correct for the patients who have had SLNB."

"What if we don't remove the node and you just follow me to see if I am the one in five or the four in five? Can't you just remove all the lymph nodes only if and when they grow big with tumor in them?"

"A metastasis in a lymph node changes your stage of the disease. It's important to know that these days because we now have effective drugs to treat you that can improve your chances of cure. If we don't know because we don't biopsy the sentinel node, the node with metastasis will eventually grow to a substantial size, and at that point, the treatment would be to remove all the nodes in the groin, and the chances of cure would drop significantly."

"What if the sentinel node is negative? Do I need the rest of the lymph nodes removed?"

"No, you don't."

"And if the sentinel node is positive, do I need the rest of the lymph nodes removed?"

"It depends upon a number of factors, including how big the metastasis in the node is and whether it is entirely within the node or has started to grow outside the node. But probably not."

"Let me get this straight. My friend told me that you removed all her groin lymph nodes because it improved the chances of cure. Now you're telling me something different."

"Yes, it is because of the development of the SLNB. The procedure was not available to her when she was treated. Now it is, and it has substantially changed the way we think about melanoma. We no longer believe that a lymphadenectomy is valuable treatment in most cases. Instead, we do SLNB as a diagnostic test. Other tests, including scans and blood tests, may be helpful, but they are not as specific and sensitive as removing the entire lymph node and looking at it under a microscope."

The operation to remove the toe melanoma and the SLNB in her left groin went well, and she never needed all her groin lymph nodes completely removed. She went back to work within a few weeks and wore normal stockings and dresses and skirts and could even go out on the tennis court without stockings and play with friends who may not have known about her melanoma.

In a time when the numbers of people in the United States diagnosed with melanoma keeps rising every year, mostly in white-skinned patients of Celtic origin, to a point where at least eighty thousand cases are diagnosed each year, often in young people, sometimes in their twenties, the potential for dying of the disease has gone down, and the number of SLNBs has risen substantially. At the same time, the number of patients that develop breast cancer is about 260,000 each year, of whom at least two hundred thousand undergo sentinel lymph node biopsies. Hundreds of thousands of people in the USA alone have avoided complete lymphadenectomies and the consequent risk of lymphedema every year for at least the last eight years. The SLNB is now the standard of care everywhere in the world, favorably affecting millions of patients.

The economics of the sentinel node era is only one aspect of the enormous impact of our pioneering studies in mice, and the vital studies of Morton and others in bringing SLNB to fruition for melanoma and breast cancer. In the US alone, the savings to the health care system and to individuals has been estimated to be at least seven billion dollars, the number rising each year.

One area where we save money is easy to understand if we look at the amount of time surgeons spend in the operating room. Health system economists tell us that it costs about $110 per minute to run an operating room. Operating time for breast cancer patients can vary depending upon many factors, but before the sentinel node era, we routinely took three to four hours per case. Now it takes about an hour and thirty minutes on the average. The downstream effect of this saved time is the ability to do more cases and take care of substantially more patients per month than was previously possible.

This is not only an advantage for breast cancer and melanoma patients, but also all the other patients from every discipline in the hospital.

Saving money by the introduction of a surgical technique can be calculated relatively easily by statisticians and economists, but there are incalculable advantages from a medical and psychological viewpoint as well. When I started my surgical training in the 1960s, patients undergoing complete lymphadenectomies for melanoma or breast cancer had to stay in the hospital for a week to ten days, mostly for pain control and management of rubber drains left in place to drain the lymph fluid from the area where the lymph nodes had been removed. As techniques and medical economics changed, those patients are often sent home after a one-night stay in the hospital. Drains have changed so much that they have suction devices and small tubes that patients can manage by themselves at home. The advantage of SLNB is patients do not need to stay in the hospital, have minimal pain, don't need drains, have smaller skin incisions, and almost no limitations of movement. They can also return to work and normal social lives much quicker than with the complete lymphadenectomy.

When cancer surgeons treating tumors other than melanoma and breast cancer saw how advantageous this might be in their own areas of expertise, they began investigating sentinel node biopsy themselves. SLNB in patients with thyroid, colon, stomach, uterus, prostate, and esophageal cancer have been successful, but there has been minimal interest by most surgeons, possibly because the techniques are not as straight forward as they are for breast cancer and melanoma. Operations on the skin and breast are two areas that are consistently easy for a good number of surgeons to learn, and patients are unlikely to go to surgeons who don't do this procedure for those conditions.

Once I had mastered the techniques of SLNB and was able to offer my expertise to patients with melanoma and breast cancer, I began to wonder how to use this information and ability to move to the next stages of lymph node management.

Chapter 22

The Metal Clip

Barbara woke up one morning, felt a lump in her left armpit, and immediately called her primary care physician who saw her the next day and sent her to me in the Multidisciplinary Breast Diagnostic Center at West Bloomfield Hospital. The advantage for patients and doctors of having a clinical facility within a radiologic breast imaging center, where surgeons and radiologists can coordinate services and see the patient on the same day, is the ability to rapidly confirm a cancer diagnosis and begin treatment as soon as possible. I was able to examine the patient, confirm that she had a suspicious lymph node in the axilla, get a mammogram immediately and an ultrasound of the axillary lump, and do needle biopsies of both the newly discovered left breast mass and the suspicious enlarged lymph node. Small metal clips were inserted into both the breast lump and the lymph node to enable us to find the area during surgery and after chemotherapy. We arranged to see her back in the clinic the following week.

The breast biopsy showed invasive breast cancer and the axillary node showed metastatic breast cancer. Her case was discussed at the Multidisciplinary Breast Cancer Tumor board by a group of specialists, and she was seen in the Breast Cancer Clinic by me and the medical oncologist on the team.

The patient was in an examining room with her husband and her daughter.

"We discussed your case with radiologists, pathologists, breast surgeons, medical oncologists, radiation oncologists, and plastic surgeons. I'm here to talk about our recommendations to treat your breast cancer. Are you comfortable with that?"

"Yes, we're fine," she said, looking at her husband and daughter.

"Do you have any questions before I begin?"

"Doctor, I want both my breasts removed."

"That is certainly an option, but I really would like to talk to you about other options before you decide."

"I want this thing out of me as soon as possible."

"I understand. Many women feel the same way. I'm interested in providing you with the best possible chance of cure, and that sometimes means using chemotherapy and targeted therapies first, before we do surgery. Can I tell you about that?"

"Do I really have to have chemotherapy at all? Can't I just have surgery and not chemo?"

"We believe you need chemotherapy, and that would be pretty standard anywhere in the country based on guidelines from the National Comprehensive Cancer Center Network. Your tumor has molecular markers that suggest it has a relatively high likelihood of spreading to internal organs. Metastases to internal organs are important because they can be life-threatening. We can do the greatest operation on the breast and armpit, but you could still get metastases. Fortunately, we have drugs that effectively kill breast cancer cells, particularly in your case because you have a HER-2 positive tumor. HER-2 is a molecule expressed in about one of every five breast cancers. There are drugs that target that molecule. When they're given intravenously, they circulate through the blood stream, bind to cells that express the molecule, and kill them. That is like a smart bomb that targets a building in enemy territory that destroys one building but leaves the buildings next to it intact. We know that about half the patients with HER-2 positive tumors given chemo plus drugs that target HER-2 will have a complete pathologic response. That means the tumor in the breast and in the lymph node is no longer visible under the microscope when we remove those tissues."

"Are you suggesting I have chemo and those other drugs first and then surgery?"

"Yes, exactly."

"Wouldn't it be better to remove the breast and the lymph node first and then use chemo?"

"Sure, we could do that. But if we do surgery first, we would have to remove not only the lymph node that has metastatic tumor in it but all the other lymph nodes in your armpit."

"Is that different to the operation you would do if I had chemo first?"

"Yes, it may be different. If you have chemo and the targeting drugs first, we could approach your axillary lymph nodes differently, trying to avert removing all the lymph nodes. We could do a targeted axillary node dissection. The radiologists placed a metal clip in that node, and instead of removing all the nodes, we would remove that lymph node and have the pathologists tell us whether there was still viable tumor in the node. If there is, we would remove the remaining nodes. But if there is no tumor in the clipped node, we could avoid going further into the axilla and leave the other nodes in you."

Her husband, an engineer by profession, was intrigued by the process, a procedure not widely known but being investigated by breast surgeons at some major cancer centers and by us.

"Can you see the clip when you operate? They showed us what it looks like when Barbara had the needle biopsies, and it seems rather tiny. And they put it in the middle of the lump."

"You're right. We can't see it with the naked eye, but we X-ray the lymph node when it is removed and that shows the clip."

"How do you know which lymph node to remove? Aren't there a bunch of them in there?"

"That's an important question. I introduced the clip idea fifteen years ago when I worked with my radiology colleagues on a research project. Do you know about sentinel node biopsy?"

They didn't know about the sentinel node, and I spent some time telling them about how we had come to the current standard of practice because we wanted to avoid lymphedema. Six years after my first SLNB in breast cancer, I had begun to believe that we might be able to avoid the operation altogether by doing a needle biopsy of the sentinel node. My radiology colleagues were a little skeptical—they wondered how we could identify the sentinel node with an ultrasound. They knew that surgeons used dyes and radiocolloid to find the correct node. But they could not use that same technique to do a needle biopsy. I suggested they concentrate on finding a lymph node at the site of the lowest axillary hair follicles, a landmark used by surgeons when making an incision in the skin at the start of an SLNB. Fortunately, despite their reluctance, my radiology colleagues helped me complete the study.

Like many of my prior research endeavors, I wrote a protocol with a hypothesis. All our new breast cancer patients gave us permission to do an ultrasound of the axilla looking for a lymph node opposite the lowest hair follicle. If there were two or more lymph nodes seen, the radiologists were to focus on the largest one, do a needle biopsy, place a metal clip through the needle, and send the tissue to the lab for analysis. The pathologist would tell us if the tissue contained lymph node structures and whether there was tumor in the node. A few days later, the patient had surgery for the breast cancer including a SLNB. When the sentinel node was removed, it was X-rayed to look for the clip and note made of the sentinel node found during surgery as being the same one with the clip in it. We found the clip in the true sentinel node in four out of five patients, published our results, and realized that we would need to continue doing SLNB in the operating room because needle biopsy was not good enough to give us the important information for staging the breast cancer. Besides, we didn't know whether removing the sentinel node could provide a greater chance of cure; if we left a lymph node containing tumor in the patient, they might not do as well as those patients in whom the node was removed.

Although there was no good reason to continue doing an ultrasound of the axilla in all our breast cancer patients, the radiologists had found a useful tool for more advanced cases, like Barbara. We realized that the likelihood of breast cancer metastasizing to the sentinel node was increased with bigger tumors, so we requested that ultrasounds be done of the axilla for breast tumors greater than two centimeters in diameter. The radiologists learned to observe which lymph nodes looked suspicious for cancer metastasis, and those were the ones they biopsied with a needle. They also felt quite comfortable leaving a clip in place.

In time it became apparent that patients with sentinel node metastasis who needed a mastectomy to treat their breast cancers might not need a complete axillary lymphadenectomy if they had a complete response of the tumor in the sentinel lymph node to chemotherapy and targeted therapy given before surgery.

"If chemo and those other drugs are so good, why do I need any surgery?" asked Barbara.

"You have a point. Unfortunately, we haven't found a reliable way to tell whether all the tumor has been killed by chemo and targeted therapy. Even MRI, the most sensitive scan currently available to look inside the breast, cannot tell us for sure that there are no viable breast cancer cells still present. If we were to leave such cells in the breast, they would grow back and be more difficult to treat."

"Is the lymph node with tumor in Barbara's armpit the sentinel lymph node?" asked Barbara's husband.

"More than likely it is. We will know when we do the SLNB. In about 10 percent of patients we X-ray, the sentinel node and the clip is not there."

"What do you do then?"

"We take out lymph nodes adjacent to the sentinel node and X-ray them until we find the clip."

"What happens if you do that and you don't find the clipped node?"

"Well, that hasn't happened yet, but I guess we might end up taking out all the axillary nodes."

"If the chemo works well, will it make the tumor in the breast much smaller? Could she have the lump removed and not the whole breast?"

"That's what we do in some cases. However, in Barbara's case, the tumor is much more extensive, and even if the mass that was biopsied goes away, there are secondary signs, such as calcium deposits, of much more extensive cancer through large areas of the breast that has not made a lump or mass. I'd love to be able to conserve her breast, but that is not safe in her case."

The patient and her family discussed the plan I had outlined with a medical oncologist, and she decided to have the chemo and targeted anti-HER-2 therapy. Ten weeks later, when I examined her again, the enlarged axillary lymph node was no longer palpable, although it was still slightly enlarged on ultrasound examination.

I did her surgery a few weeks later. The sentinel node was slightly firm, which often means cancer is still present, although sometimes after chemo the tumor may be gone and in its place is scar tissue, which can also be firm. The pathologist found tumor in the node, and we proceeded to remove all of the rest of her axillary lymph nodes. Only one out of nineteen lymph nodes showed evidence of breast cancer. My plastic surgery colleague did a breast reconstruction and a lympho-venous anastomosis, a new procedure designed to connect severed lymphatics to veins with the hope that the chances of developing lymphedema would be diminished.

The targeted axillary lymphadenectomy which we did on Barbara did not help her, but I have had several patients who had this procedure who managed to avoid a complete axillary lymphadenectomy. It is still too early to tell, but my introduction of the metal clip into a metastatic lymph node, based on a sound original idea, provided enough new information to use the clip to advance another new lymph node operation that will likely save many women the agony of getting lymphedema of the arm.

This was another simple idea that provided an impetus to develop a better approach to breast cancer treatment which arose simply by thinking through the next phase of development.

Chapter 23

Concealed Until It Is Revealed

Medical students can initiate ideas, and Krasnick and Arbabi, two third-year students from Wayne State Medical School assigned to help me with patients in the operating room, were hungry for research projects.

"I heard you have a number of research projects, and I'd love to get involved," said Brad.

The three of us met the next day in my clinic, and I shared data from one of my latest studies that showed breast cancer in the sentinel lymph node caused an increase in pressure in the node; the size of the metastasis in millimeters directly related to the pressure measured during the operation to remove the node. This observation had confirmed my hypothesis, but I had questions related to the measurement of the tumor size. I had often wondered about the relationship of the volume of tumor and the pressure in breast cancer. The measurement here was based upon caliper measurement from one side of the tumor in the lymph node to the other by a pathologist and was reported as such in the pathology report.

"I'm looking to determine whether we can relate the size of the tumor to the volume of the lymph node that houses the metastasis," I said. "If you guys are interested, you could take the data from this study and calculate the volume of the sentinel node. The pathologists provide a measurement of the length, breadth, and width of the node, and you could calculate the volume of each node, compare that to the reported size of the metastasis in the node, do a statistical analysis, and we could publish a paper."

They were both excited about the project.

"Okay, great," I said. "The first issue is to create an appropriate formula for calculating the volume of a lymph node. If it were a cylinder you could take the height and radius and use a simple formula, $V = r^2 h$, and have an accurate volume. For a sphere, the formula is $V = 4/3 \, \pi r^3$. For a cube, it is $V = a^3$. I don't know what the correct formula would be for a lymph node which is shaped like a kidney bean, but you can ask one of the physicists at Wayne or in radiation physics."

Both the guys worked hard and gave the completed numbers to the statistician. The analysis showed that the volume of the sentinel node increased proportionate to the size of the metastasis, a conclusion which complemented the deductions which clinicians had been teaching for decades that lymph nodes that are enlarged and hard usual harbor metastases. Our study was the first to accurately measure the volume of the sentinel lymph node and relate it directly to the size of the metastasis. Clinicians are taught to observe and record objectively but crudely what they see, smell, touch, hear, taste, and compare, a phenomenon in clinical medicine going back centuries. In contrast, trained observers in some other professions, like physics, are more likely to use the most accurate tool for measuring and comparing.

It was time to report the results, and Brad, alert and respectful but also anxious to heighten his chances of getting into the best surgical training programs in the country, came to me to ask if he could present the data at the annual San Antonio Breast Cancer Symposium.

"Brad, I usually present the paper when I produce the original idea and do the experiment. I would normally put your and Arbabi's name on the paper because you did a lot of the leg work, but I would be the first author. In this case, I love your enthusiasm and assistance so much that I want you to take this study as far as you can. Presenting a paper like this at an international meeting of such high quality as a medical student would be a fabulous way to kickstart your post-graduate career. When you interview for positions at major general surgery programs around the country, the final decision between you and a rival might be tilted by this research project."

He was delighted, and the paper was accepted, and he presented it, and two years later, when he was in training at the prestigious Washington University in St. Louis, he wrote and published the full paper with Arbabi, who was also training in General Surgery in a prominent training program in California, as a co-author.

The world is full of concealed things. Krasnick and Arbabi's talent at completing a research project was concealed until they came forward and showed their enthusiasm and exercised their curiosity. They are part of the generation that will hopefully take over from my generation, teaching the next generation, who will teach the generation after that. Each new generation will think about new ideas, ideas that would remain concealed without their energy, curiosity, and hard work to improve the world.

The sentinel lymph node was always there, although concealed, as were many things discovered by people with ideas and the energy to investigate those ideas. The sentinel node was concealed, and it was only revealed by the imagination of several people whose ideas have been described in this book. We might have managed to continue treating breast cancer and melanoma with the operation of complete lymphadenectomy, and patients may have been cured as frequently as they are now but with severe complications, such as lymphedema. This is analogous to useful navigation techniques used by pre-Copernican/Galilean sailors who believed the planets and the sun revolve around the earth; they could still navigate and explore the earth without getting lost. However, space travel would not have been possible without the Heliocentric astronomical model, a new understanding based on science. So, too, advances in the surgical management of BC and melanoma in the future will depend upon improved understanding of the mechanisms by which tumors metastasize to sentinel lymph nodes and systemic sites.

SLN biopsy has had a dramatic impact on the accuracy of staging in melanoma and breast cancer, and the presence of metastatic tumor in the SLN is one of the most powerful predictors of how well the patient will do in the future, independent of other known factors, although there are many other factors in the patient and in the tumor that are important in determining the patient's outcome. SLN biopsy is now known to be better than other less invasive technologies for finding tumor in lymph nodes, such as ultrasound.

Innovation and adaptation will be necessary for continued relevance of SLN biopsy, which will likely take place in several areas. There would need to be incremental advances helping to optimize an already good technique. Other avenues of research could advance SLN utility even further, including developing more refined criteria for selecting patients for SLN biopsy. Some advances may make SLN biopsy redundant; for example, we can imagine non-surgical therapies that will kill tumor in lymph nodes in which case removing them might become unnecessary. We still don't know for certain whether removing the SLN treats melanoma and breast cancer and that will require further research.

The era of the sentinel node has exposed areas of research in the immune reaction to melanoma and other cancers since the SLN is the first site of interaction of a melanoma with the immune system. The nature of this interaction may provide insights about the nature of the body's antitumor response and enlighten us as to how tumors protect themselves from the body's immune system. New therapies will likely emerge, eventually making our current approaches to cancers antiquated, much like modern nuclear weapons make knights in armor on horseback quite ludicrous. Until such technologies materialize and mature, the identification of early sentinel lymph node metastasis in patients with clinically localized melanoma and breast cancer is one of the best biomarkers available to inform clinicians and patients of the possibility of cure and will continue to guide treatment, and the SLN technique will likely remain a central part of patient care for the foreseeable future.

We also must investigate other areas of knowledge which are currently concealed but which we imagine are important. Amongst those currently hidden from view are how tumor cells communicate and interact with each other using molecules that we have not yet found and with the tumor micro-environment, the extracellular matrix and the immune system. New knowledge is inevitable since we can never claim to have revealed everything there is to know; but we will only discover and understand if we continue to search hard for the hidden truths.

My hope is that we will forever cultivate the imagination and questions of the young in our societies, keep encouraging their advances with an open mind, be open to investigating new ideas, accept that old methodologies may need to be supplanted by new ones, and encourage the passion of discovery.

That's what happened to me.

CPSIA information can be obtained
at www.ICGtesting.com
Printed in the USA
LVHW061812280421
685611LV00014BA/661/J